Annual Review of Eating Disorders Part 2 – 2006

Edited by
Stephen Wonderlich
James E Mitchell
Martina de Zwaan
Howard Steiger

Foreword by
Scott J Crow

RADCLIFFE PUBLISHING
OXFORD • SEATTLE

Radcliffe Publishing Ltd
18 Marcham Road
Abingdon
Oxon OX14 1AA
United Kingdom

www.radcliffe-oxford.com
Electronic catalogue and worldwide online ordering facility.

British Library Cataloguing in Publication Data

A catalogue record for this book is available from the British Library.

ISBN-10 1 84619 020 7
ISBN-13 978 1 84619 020 9

Typeset by Advance Typesetting Ltd, Oxford
Printed and bound by TJ International Ltd, Padstow, Cornwall

Contents

Foreword

The field of eating disorders (EDs) is rapidly evolving and developing. The recent research contributions to the field described in this book are ample evidence of the rapid progress being made towards understanding the causes, complications, course, treatment, and prevention of EDs. As the amount of this work continues to increase (and the forums in which it is published continue to broaden), the task of keeping up to date on this growing literature becomes all the more difficult.

This *Annual Review of Eating Disorders Part 2 – 2006* represents a wonderful solution to this problem, and is a thoughtful and thorough review of recent progress in the field. This review is a particular point of pride for the Academy for Eating Disorders (AED) and is a clear expression of the Academy's professional education mission. This volume represents the completion of the two-year cycle of reviews. Thus, next year's Annual Review will cover another two years of progress on the topics reviewed in the first edition. Last year's Review was extremely well received, and I am confident the same will be true this year.

As current President for the Academy for Eating Disorders I extend my thanks to Stephen Wonderlich, James Mitchell, Martina de Zwaan, and Howard Steiger for their outstanding efforts as editors, and to each of the individual authors of chapters in this volume.

Scott J Crow, MD
President, Academy for Eating Disorders
September 2005

List of editors

Stephen Wonderlich, PhD
Neuropsychiatric Research Institute and Department of Clinical Neuroscience,
University of North Dakota School of Medicine and Health Sciences, Fargo,
USA

James E Mitchell, MD
Neuropsychiatric Research Institute and Department of Clinical Neuroscience,
University of North Dakota School of Medicine and Health Sciences, Fargo,
USA

Martina de Zwaan, MD
University of Erlangen, Erlangen, Germany

Howard Steiger, PhD
Douglas Hospital, McGill University, Montreal, Canada

List of contributors

Emily L Ach
Department of Psychology, Wesleyan University, Middletown, CT

Ursula F Bailer, MD
University of Pittsburgh School of Medicine, Department of Psychiatry, Western Psychiatric Institute and Clinic, Pittsburgh, PA
Medical University of Vienna, Department of General Psychiatry, University Hospital of Psychiatry, Vienna, Austria

Anne E Becker, MD, PhD, ScM
Department of Psychiatry, Massachusetts General Hospital
Department of Social Medicine, Harvard Medical School

Rachel J Bryant-Waugh, MSc, DPhil
University of Southampton and Hampshire Partnership NHS Trust, UK

Cynthia M Bulik
Department of Psychiatry, University of North Carolina at Chapel Hill

Christopher G Fairburn
Oxford University Department of Psychiatry, Warneford Hospital, Oxford, UK

Kristen Fay, BA
Eliot-Pearson Department of Applied Clinical Development, Tufts University, Boston, MA

Guido Frank, MD
University of California San Diego, School of Medicine, Department of Child and Adolescent Psychiatry, San Diego, CA
California University of Pittsburgh School of Medicine, Department of Psychiatry, Western Psychiatric Institute and Clinic, Pittsburgh, PA

Debra L Franko
Department of Counseling and Applied Educational Psychology, Northeastern University, Boston, MA

Katherine A Halmi, MD
Weill Cornell Medical College, White Plains, NY

Leslie J Heinberg, PhD
Department of Epidemiology and Biostatistics, Case Western Reserve University, Cleveland, OH

David C Jimerson, MD
Department of Psychiatry, Beth Israel Deaconess Medical Center and Harvard Medical School, Boston, MA

Walter H Kaye, MD
University of Pittsburgh, School of Medicine, Department of Psychiatry, Western Psychiatric Institute and Clinic, Pittsburgh, PA

Suzanne E Mazzeo, PhD
Departments of Psychology and Pediatrics, Virginia Commonwealth University, Richmond, VA

Joanna Peart, BA
Department of Psychology, Emory University, Atlanta, GA

Margarita CT Slof-Op't Landt
National Centre for Eating Disorders, Leidschendam/Oegstgeest, The Netherlands

Ruth H Striegel-Moore
Department of Psychology, Wesleyan University, Middletown, CT

J Kevin Thompson, PhD
Department of Psychology, University of South Florida, Tampa, FL

Heather Thompson-Brenner, PhD
Center for Anxiety and Related Disorders, Boston University, Boston, MA

Eric F van Furth
National Centre for Eating Disorders, Leidschendam/Oegstgeest, The Netherlands

Angela Wagner, MD
University of Pittsburgh, School of Medicine, Department of Psychiatry, Western Psychiatric Institute and Clinic, Pittsburgh, PA
JW Goethe University of Frankfurt/main. Department of Child and Adolescent Psychiatry, Frankfurt, Germany

Drew Westen, PhD
Departments of Psychology and Psychiatry and Behavioral Sciences, Emory University, Atlanta, GA

Barbara E Wolfe, PhD
Connell School of Nursing, Boston College, Chestnut Hill, MA

1

Psychobiology of eating disorders

David C Jimerson and Barbara E Wolfe

Abstract

Objectives of review. The goal of this review is to highlight selected advances during 2003–2004 in research on the psychobiology of the eating disorders.

Summary of recent findings. Studies in bulimia nervosa (BN) have demonstrated associations between alterations in serotonin function and comorbid psychiatric disorders, while studies in both BN and anorexia nervosa (AN) have provided additional evidence for persistent, possibly trait-related alterations in serotonin regulation. Studies of leptin function have shown an association between circulating levels of the protein and symptom patterns during the course of recovery from AN. Studies of ghrelin function have provided new evidence for altered postprandial release of the peptide in BN and binge-eating disorder, and elevated baseline levels of the peptide in AN.

Future directions. Additional research will be needed to assess both categorical and dimensional clinical correlates of alterations in these neurobiological systems. Studies in individuals who have recovered from the eating disorders will be valuable in identifying stable psychobiological characteristics. Future results may lead to new pharmacological treatment approaches.

Introduction

A variety of factors have contributed to the rapid acceleration of research on the psychobiology of eating disorders. Preclinical advances in molecular and behavioral neurobiology have led to increased understanding of the regulation of neurotransmitters, neuropeptides, neurohormones and other neuromodulators acting in the hypothalamus and cortical brain regions to regulate food intake, mood, stress response and cognition. Preclinical and clinical investigations related to obesity and energy metabolism have led to increased understanding of the important role of peripheral signals, particularly involving gut peptides and adipokines, in influencing central nervous system (CNS) processes regulating energy metabolism and eating patterns. New technologies for clinical investigation, including functional imaging and genetics, have also accelerated the pace of research. Finally, there has been increased refinement of diagnostic criteria and more detailed understanding of symptom patterns associated with the eating disorders.

The current review focuses selectively on the neurotransmitter serotonin, the adipokine leptin, and the gut-related peptide ghrelin. These neurobiological messengers appear likely to play an important role in our understanding of the eating disorders, and have been the focus of intensive study during the period of 2003 to 2004 covered by the review. Within each section, we provide a brief overview of studies through 2002, and a more focused outline of new research during the review period. Related aspects of research advances, particularly with regard to serotonin function, are reviewed in the chapters on 'Review of brain imaging in anorexia and bulimia nervosa' and 'Genetics of eating disorders'.

Literature review

Serotonin

Interest in the possible role of abnormal serotonin regulation in the eating disorders has been driven by preclinical studies showing that serotonin plays an important role in regulating meal patterns; by clinical studies associating serotonin with symptoms of depression, impulsivity and obsessive-compulsive behavioral patterns; and by research indicating that therapeutic effects of antidepressant medications are associated with augmentation of synaptic serotonin function (Wolfe *et al.* 1997). Of particular interest are recent studies showing that serotonin interacts with other neurotransmitters and neuropeptides in the hypothalamus to regulate eating behavior (Heisler *et al.* 2003).

Serotonin function in bulimia nervosa

As previously reviewed (Wolfe *et al.* 1997; Kaye *et al.* 2004), BN appears to be associated with a decrease in CNS serotonin function. Thus, in comparison to healthy controls, patients with BN have decreased concentration of the serotonin metabolite 5-hydroxyindoleacetic acid (5-HIAA) in cerebrospinal fluid (CSF), and blunted neuroendocrine responses to serotonin agonist drugs such as m-chlorophenylpiperazine (mCPP) or fenfluramine. Other evidence for altered serotonin regulation in BN emerged from studies of acute tryptophan depletion (Kaye *et al.* 2000) and platelet antidepressant (e.g. $[^3H]$-paroxetine) binding (Steiger *et al.* 2001a).

Several groups have explored the relationship between binge-eating behavior, comorbid psychiatric symptomatology and serotonergic responsiveness. In CSF metabolite and neuroendocrine studies, patients with the highest severity of bulimic symptoms have shown the most prominent deficit in serotonergic responses (Jimerson *et al.* 1997; Monteleone *et al.* 2000). In a series of studies, Steiger and colleagues reported that alterations in serotonergic neuroendocrine and platelet measures in patients with BN appeared to be associated with a range of behavioral characteristics (Steiger 2004), including childhood abuse (Steiger *et al.* 2004), self-destructiveness (Steiger *et al.* 2001b), impulsivity (Steiger *et al.* 2003) and avoidant personality (Bruce *et al.* 2004). Another recent study found that platelet paroxetine binding was altered in patients with AN or BN, although the platelet measures did not appear to be correlated with symptom severity, impulsivity or depression (Ramacciotti *et al.* 2003). Relatively small samples for BN in the latter study may, however, have provided limited power for detecting associations between neurobiological and symptom indices. In addition, the effects of severe malnutrition in patients with AN may limit the ability to detect underlying associations between peripheral neurobiological indices and behavioral traits.

Functional imaging studies using single-photon emission computed tomography (SPECT) or positron emission tomography (PET) in BN have shown, in comparison to controls, regional decreases in brain serotonin transporter availability (Tauscher *et al.* 2001) and increases in 5-HT_{1A} receptor binding (Tiihonen *et al.* 2004), but no apparent alteration in binding to the 5HT_{2A} receptor (Goethals *et al.* 2004).

There has been considerable interest in whether or not there are trait-related alterations in serotonin function in individuals with a history of BN following remission of abnormal eating patterns. Findings to date indicate that recovered individuals have elevated levels of CSF 5-HIAA, increased sensitivity to reduction of serotonin synthesis following acute tryptophan depletion, and regional decreases in 5-HT_{2A} binding, but apparently normal neuroendocrine responses (Kaye *et al.* 1998; Smith *et al.* 1999; Wolfe *et al.* 2000; Kaye *et al.* 2001).

Serotonin function in binge-eating disorder

An initial study reported normal neuroendocrine responses to a serotonin agonist drug in patients with this disorder (Monteleone *et al.* 2000). Of interest, obese patients with binge eating were shown to have reduced serotonin transporter binding (as measured by SPECT) in comparison to obese controls (Kuikka *et al.* 2001). Transporter binding was found to increase in symptomatically recovered patients (Tammela *et al.* 2003).

Serotonin function in anorexia nervosa

Studies in AN have consistently shown reduced serotonin function, as reflected in significant reduction of 5-HIAA concentration in CSF and diminished neuro-endocrine response to serotonergic agonist drugs (Brewerton and Jimerson 1996; Wolfe *et al.* 1997; Kaye *et al.* 2004). A brain imaging study using SPECT demon-strated regional cortical reduction in 5-HT_{2A} binding (Audenaert *et al.* 2003). Given that dieting and weight loss can have substantial effects on CNS serotonin, it is difficult to ascertain the extent to which these alterations in low-weight patients bear a specific relationship to the eating disorder and to what extent they reflect non-specific effects of nutritional deprivation.

To control for nutritional effects, several groups have studied patients as they reached goal weight during treatment, and in general, results showed a tendency for serotonin function to return towards normal (Brewerton *et al.* 1996). How-ever, following short-term weight restoration some patients still show altered behavioral responses to a serotonergic drug (Frank *et al.* 2001).

There has been considerable interest in studies comparing long-term weight recovered patients with healthy controls matched for body mass index (BMI). Results have shown elevated levels of CSF 5-HIAA (Kaye *et al.* 1991) and diminished sensitivity to the behavioral effects of fenfluramine (Ward *et al.* 1998), although neuroendocrine responses are not different from healthy controls (O'Dwyer *et al.* 1996). Moreover, acute tryptophan depletion resulted in a decrease in symptoms of anxiety in long-term recovered individuals (Kaye *et al.* 2003). Persistent alteration of serotonin function following remission is reflected in the finding that regional 5-HT_{2A} receptor binding is decreased in individuals who have recovered from the binge-eating/purging subtype of AN (Bailer *et al.* 2004).

Leptin

In the decade since the discovery of the *ob (Lep)* gene, there has been increased understanding of the role of leptin in bodyweight regulation. In humans as in laboratory animals, serum and CSF leptin levels show a robust correlation with body fat content and with BMI (Mantzoros *et al.* 1997; Friedman 2000). Leptin acts in the CNS to decrease meal size and food intake, with interactions in the hypothalamus involving neuropeptide Y, the melanocortins and the neuro-transmitter serotonin (Zigman and Elmquist 2003). It is of note that leptin plays a role in brain development in hypothalamic circuits involved in regulation of eating behavior (Elmquist and Flier 2004).

Leptin in bulimia nervosa

As recently reviewed (Monteleone *et al.* 2004), studies comparing serum leptin levels in patients with BN have generally reported lower levels than in healthy controls matched for BMI. The decrease in leptin levels is most apparent in patients with the most severe symptomatology (Jimerson *et al.* 2000; Monteleone *et al.* 2002). These findings are consistent with the hypothesis that low leptin in BN contributes to binge eating and reduced metabolic rate. However, other studies comparing baseline leptin levels in patients with BN and controls have reported variable results, possibly as a result of heterogeneity in patient populations and the inclusion of less symptomatic patients than in the earlier studies (Calandra *et al.* 2003; Monteleone *et al.* 2003b; Tagami *et al.* 2004; Housova *et al.* 2005). Another possible confounding factor is the finding that leptin levels decrease during short periods of caloric deficit prior to a significant change in body composition (Chin-Chance *et al.* 2000). Additionally, healthy volunteers following a reduced calorie diet over several weeks show a marked decrease in serum leptin levels (Wolfe *et al.* 2004). Thus, future studies comparing eating disorder patients with controls will benefit from efforts to monitor the stability of caloric intake over the days preceding study.

An initial report did not demonstrate a significant difference between leptin levels in individuals who had recovered from BN and healthy controls (Gendall *et al.* 1999). However, a subsequent study which was adjusted for body fat percentage found significantly reduced leptin levels in individuals recovered from the eating disorder (Jimerson *et al.* 2000).

Leptin in binge-eating disorder

Some studies of patients with binge-eating disorder have shown elevated leptin levels when compared with overweight controls matched for BMI (d'Amore *et al.* 2001; Adami *et al.* 2002), while other reports have shown no significant difference (Monteleone *et al.* 2002; Geliebter *et al.* 2004). Future studies may help to clarify these variable findings by matching subjects for eating patterns prior to study, as well as for BMI and percentage of body fat.

Leptin in anorexia nervosa

Serum and CSF leptin concentrations in patients with AN are markedly lower than in healthy, normal weight controls, as recently reviewed (Monteleone *et al.* 2004). Given that circulating leptin levels are substantially influenced by body fat content, low leptin levels in this disorder are most likely a consequence of malnutrition. A substantial portion of serum total leptin is bound to a circulating form of the soluble leptin receptor, with evidence that free (unbound) leptin plays an important role in leptin action (Zastrow *et al.* 2003). Circulating levels of the binding protein are elevated in patients with AN, resulting in a markedly diminished free leptin index (Kratzsch *et al.* 2002; Krizova *et al.* 2002; Monteleone *et al.* 2002; Misra *et al.* 2004a). Leptin levels increase with weight restoration in patients with AN and, following long-term recovery, serum and CSF leptin levels appear to be not significantly different from control values (Gendall *et al.* 1999; Brown *et al.* 2003; Popovic *et al.* 2004).

Several lines of investigation suggest that the marked reduction in circulating leptin in AN may contribute to physiological and behavioral symptoms. Administration of leptin to rodents can suppress hyperactivity (Exner *et al.* 2000), and clinical studies have shown an association between hyperactivity in AN and low serum leptin levels (Hebebrand *et al.* 2003; Holtkamp *et al.* 2003b). Preclinical and clinical observations indicate that decreased leptin in AN may contribute to amenorrhea (Holtkamp *et al.* 2003c; Ahima and Osei, 2004). It is of interest that patients who have achieved weight restoration but have persistent amenorrhea show significantly lower serum leptin levels, as well as reduced estrogen levels, in comparison to controls (Brambilla *et al.* 2003; Popovic *et al.* 2004). Additionally, low leptin levels may play a role in the osteopenia associated with AN (Miller *et al.* 2004).

During weight restoration, serum leptin levels return to a normal range before patients reach a normal BMI (Mantzoros *et al.* 1997; Holtkamp *et al.* 2003a). This finding has led to the hypothesis that an overshoot in leptin levels could contribute to resistance to full weight restoration (Mantzoros *et al.* 1997), and to the notably increased metabolic rate associated with refeeding (Hebebrand *et al.* 1997). One study suggested that elevated serum leptin levels at the time of discharge from an inpatient treatment program may be associated with less favorable clinical outcome over the ensuing year (Holtkamp *et al.* 2004). However, another study which attempted to adjust the rate of weight gain to minimize overshoot in serum leptin levels was unable to show significantly improved outcome (Lob *et al.* 2003).

In addition to leptin, other adipokines may play a role in the eating disorders. Adiponectin, for example, is a protein that is released from adipose tissue and has an effect of enhancing insulin sensitivity and improving lipid metabolism (Diez and Iglesias 2003). Initial studies have reported variable findings for adiponectin in BN (Monteleone *et al.* 2003a; Tagami *et al.* 2004), and decreased levels in binge-eating disorder (Monteleone *et al.* 2003a). Consistent with an inverse correlation between adiponectin and BMI (Arita *et al.* 1999), most studies to date indicate that adiponectin levels are increased in AN (Delporte *et al.* 2003; Iwahashi *et al.* 2003; Pannacciulli *et al.* 2003), although low values have also been reported (Tagami *et al.* 2004).

Ghrelin

Increasing understanding of the role that gut-related peptides play in the regulation of meal patterns has led to hypotheses that the binge episodes of BN might be related to impaired release of peptides that enhance satiety and limit meal size, or to excessive release of peptides that normally promote hunger and increase meal size. Thus, as recently reviewed (Jimerson and Wolfe 2004), it has been of interest that postprandial release of the satiety-promoting gut peptide cholecystokinin (CCK) is diminished in BN. (Results for postprandial CCK release in AN have been more variable (Jimerson *et al.* 2004; Tomasik *et al.* 2004).) Recent findings raise the possibility that alterations in gastric capacity or gastric function in BN and binge-eating disorder could contribute to abnormalities in the release of peptides from the gastrointestinal tract (Geliebter and Hashim 2001; Walsh *et al.* 2003).

Ghrelin is a gut-related peptide which has received substantial research attention during the 2003–2004 period. Initially identified as a circulating stimulator of growth hormone release (Neary *et al.* 2003), ghrelin is released from endocrine cells of the stomach and acts in the hypothalamus to increase meal size (Chen *et al.* 2004). Administration of ghrelin to healthy volunteers increases meal size and hunger ratings (Wren *et al.* 2001). Fasting, diet-induced weight loss and gastric bypass surgery have been associated with an increase in ghrelin levels in the blood (Cummings *et al.* 2002; Leidy *et al.* 2004).

Ghrelin in bulimia nervosa

Studies of baseline plasma ghrelin levels in BN have yielded variable results. Initial reports indicated that in patients with the purging subtype of BN studied after overnight fast, circulating ghrelin levels were significantly higher than for healthy controls matched for BMI (Tanaka *et al.* 2002, 2003a; Kojima *et al.* 2005). Additionally, ghrelin levels were positively correlated with the frequency of binge/purge episodes, while the levels in the non-purging type of the disorder were not significantly different from control values. However, another report indicated that ghrelin levels measured after overnight fast in patients with the purging type of BN were not significantly different from control values, and were not correlated with the frequency of binge/purge episodes (Monteleone *et al.* 2005). Ghrelin levels measured at midday were not significantly different for patients with BN and controls (Monteleone *et al.* 2003b; Nakazato *et al.* 2004).

In healthy volunteers, ghrelin levels decrease markedly following a meal. The ghrelin response to a standardized meal is significantly attenuated in patients with BN in comparison to controls (Monteleone *et al.* 2003b; Kojima *et al.* 2005). This finding is consistent with the observation of impaired postingestive satiety in BN, and suggests that abnormal ghrelin regulation could contribute to the large amount of food consumed during binge-eating episodes.

Ghrelin in binge-eating disorder

Baseline plasma ghrelin levels in patients with binge-eating disorder were significantly lower than values for normal weight controls, but not significantly different from levels found in obese non-binge-eating subjects (Geliebter *et al.* 2004; Monteleone *et al.* 2005). Similar to findings in bulimia nervosa, subjects with binge-eating disorder showed a blunted decrease in postprandial ghrelin levels.

Ghrelin in anorexia nervosa

Circulating ghrelin levels in patients with AN are significantly elevated in comparison to healthy controls (Otto *et al.* 2001; Rigamonti *et al.* 2002; Shiiya *et al.* 2002; Krsek *et al.* 2003; Nedvídková *et al.* 2003; Tanaka *et al.* 2003a; Broglio *et al.*

2004; Misra *et al.* 2004b; Soriano-Guillén *et al.* 2004; Stock *et al.* 2005). Moreover, plasma ghrelin levels in women with AN were significantly elevated in comparison to constitutionally thin women who were studied at a similar BMI (although the latter subjects had a significantly higher percentage of fat mass than the patient group) (Tolle *et al.* 2003). As patients regain weight their plasma ghrelin levels decrease towards normal values (Otto *et al.* 2001; Tolle *et al.* 2003; Soriano-Guillén *et al.* 2004; Tanaka *et al.* 2004). It has been reported that patients of the binge-eating/purging subtype of AN have higher plasma ghrelin levels than patients of the restricting type (Tanaka *et al.* 2003a,b), although this difference was not observed by others (Otto *et al.* 2004).

Studies of total ghrelin concentration in plasma reflect both acylated (or intact) ghrelin, which is thought to be the biologically active form of the peptide, as well as desacyl (or degraded) ghrelin, which may also have some biological activity (Akamizu *et al.* 2005; Inui 2005). An initial study reported that active ghrelin was elevated in five patients with AN in comparison to seven normal controls (Nakai *et al.* 2003). However, another study measuring intact ghrelin in patients with AN found that these levels were either lower than or similar to control values, based on two different assay methods, while levels of the degraded forms of ghrelin were elevated in the patient group (Hotta *et al.* 2004). These authors speculated that elevated levels of degraded ghrelin in AN could result from decreased renal clearance associated with dehydration and malnutrition.

The postprandial decrease in plasma ghrelin in AN has been reported as blunted (Nedvídková *et al.* 2003), or similar to control values (Stock *et al.* 2005). Following oral glucose administration, one study showed robust suppression of active ghrelin in patients with AN (Nakai *et al.* 2003), another study showed suppression of total ghrelin (Misra *et al.* 2004b), while another study reported a delayed time course of ghrelin suppression (Tanaka *et al.* 2003c). Following intravenous glucose administration, patients with the disorder showed a significant decrease in active ghrelin, but not in degraded ghrelin (Hotta *et al.* 2004). Follow-up studies will be needed to help clarify the relationships between total ghrelin, active ghrelin and degraded ghrelin in AN, and the relationship of peptide levels to clinical symptom patterns.

Summary of important findings

As noted in the introduction, the goal of this selective review has been to highlight recent advances in several promising areas of research on the psychobiology of the eating disorders. Studies of serotonin function suggest that this neurotransmitter system plays a role in the symptoms of BN and AN, and that persisting, possibly trait-related, changes may reflect a biological vulnerability factor for the development of these disorders. Alterations in leptin levels may contribute to symptom patterns in patients with AN at low weight and during weight restoration. Diminished ghrelin responses to a meal in BN and in binge-eating disorder may play a role in impaired postingestive satiety and the tendency for binge episodes.

Clinical implications

Accumulating evidence from physiological, brain imaging, pharmacological and genetic studies indicates that neurobiological characteristics are likely to play a role in the onset or persistence of the eating disorders, and may contribute to the risk for relapse following recovery. With additional research, these findings are likely to lead to the development of new approaches to treatment, and to preventive interventions for individuals at increased risk for developing an eating disorder.

Future directions

Additional research will be needed to assess diagnostic (categorical), dimensional and symptomatic correlates of alterations in neurobiological function. Studies in individuals who have recovered from the eating disorders will be important in identifying stable psychobiological characteristics likely to be independent of illness-related alterations in nutrition and bodyweight. Dynamic studies evaluating physiological responses to dietary alterations, test-meals and cognitive challenges will be informative. Additional studies of pilot interventions (e.g. involving the serotonin system) may provide the basis for larger clinical trials.

Acknowledgments

Supported in part by USPHS grant R01 MH45466 (DCJ) and the Bernice S Weisman Fund.

Corresponding author: David C Jimerson, MD, Department of Psychiatry, Beth Israel Deaconess Medical Center and Harvard Medical School, 330 Brookline Avenue, Boston, MA 02215, USA. Email: djimerso@bidmc.Harvard.edu

References

References preceded by three asterisks are of particular significance. The significance is explained by a short commentary following the complete reference.

Adami G, Campostano A, Cella F and Ferrandes G (2002) Serum leptin level and restrained eating: study with the Eating Disorder Examination. *Physiol Behav*, 75: 189–92.

Ahima RS and Osei SY (2004) Leptin signaling. *Physiol Behav*, 81: 223–41.

Akamizu T, Shinomiya T, Irako T, Fukunaga M, Nakai Y, Nakai Y et al. (2005) Separate measurement of plasma levels of acylated and desacyl ghrelin in healthy subjects using a new direct ELISA assay. *J Clin Endocrinol Metab*, 90: 6–9.

Arita Y, Kihara S, Ouchi N, Takahashi M, Maeda K, Miyagawa J et al. (1999) Paradoxical decrease of an adipose-specific protein, adiponectin, in obesity. *Biochem Biophys Res Commun*, 257: 79–83.

Audenaert K, Van Laere K, Dumont F, Vervaet M, Goethals I, Slegers G *et al.* (2003) Decreased 5-HT2a receptor binding in patients with anorexia nervosa. *J Nucl Med*, **44**: 163–9.

Bailer UF, Price JC, Meltzer CC, Mathis CA, Frank GK, Weissfeld L *et al.* (2004) Altered 5-HT(2A) receptor binding after recovery from bulimia-type anorexia nervosa: relationships to harm avoidance and drive for thinness. *Neuropsychopharmacology*, **89**: 1143–55.

Brambilla F, Monteleone P, Bortolotti F, Dalle GR, Todisco P, Favaro A *et al.* (2003) Persistent amenorrhoea in weight–recovered anorexics: psychological and biological aspects. *Psychiatry Res*, **118**: 249–57.

Brewerton TD and Jimerson DC (1996) Studies of serotonin function in anorexia nervosa. *Psychiatry Res*, **89**: 31–42.

Broglio F, Gianotti L, Destefanis S, Fassino S, Abbate DG, Mondelli V *et al.* (2004) The endocrine response to acute ghrelin administration is blunted in patients with anorexia nervosa, a ghrelin hypersecretory state. *Clin Endocrinol (Oxf)*, **89**: 592–9.

Brown NW, Ward A, Surwit R, Tiller J, Lightman S, Treasure JL *et al.* (2003) Evidence for metabolic and endocrine abnormalities in subjects recovered from anorexia nervosa. *Metabolism*, **89**: 296–302.

Bruce KR, Steiger H, Koerner NM, Israel M and Young SN (2004) Bulimia nervosa with co-morbid avoidant personality disorder: behavioral characteristics and serotonergic function. *Psychol Med*, **89**: 113–24.

Calandra C, Musso F and Musso R (2003) The role of leptin in the etiopathogenesis of anorexia nervosa and bulimia. *Eat Weight Disord*, **8**: 130–7.

Chen HY, Trumbauer ME, Chen AS, Weingarth DT, Adams JR, Frazier EG *et al.* (2004) Orexigenic action of peripheral ghrelin is mediated by neuropeptide Y and agouti-related protein. *Endocrinology*, **145**: 2607–12.

Chin-Chance C, Polonsky KS and Schoeller DA (2000) Twenty-four-hour leptin levels respond to cumulative short-term energy imbalance and predict subsequent intake. *J Clin Endocrinol Metab*, **89**: 2685–91.

Cummings DE, Weigle DS, Frayo RS, Breen PA, Ma MK, Dellinger EP *et al.* (2002) Plasma ghrelin levels after diet-induced weight loss or gastric bypass surgery. *N Engl J Med*, **346**: 1623–30.

d'Amore A, Massignan C, Montera P, Moles A, De Lorenzo A and Scucchi S (2001) Relationship between dietary restraint, binge eating, and leptin in obese women. *Int J Obes Relat Metab Disord*, **89**: 373–7.

Delporte ML, Brichard SM, Hermans MP, Beguin C and Lambert M (2003) Hyperadiponectinaemia in anorexia nervosa. *Clin Endocrinol (Oxf)*, **89**: 22–9.

Diez JJ and Iglesias P (2003) The role of the novel adipocyte-derived hormone adiponectin in human disease. *Eur J Endocrinol*, **148**: 293–300.

Elmquist JK and Flier JS (2004) Neuroscience. The fat–brain axis enters a new dimension. *Science*, **304**: 63–4.

Exner C, Hebebrand J, Remschmidt H, Wewetzer C, Ziegler A, Herpertz S *et al.* (2000) Leptin suppresses semi-starvation induced hyperactivity in rats: implications for anorexia nervosa. *Mol Psychiatry*, **5**: 476–81.

Frank GK, Kaye WH, Weltzin TE, Perel J, Moss H, McConaha C *et al.* (2001) Altered response to meta-chlorophenylpiperazine in anorexia nervosa: support for a persistent alteration of serotonin activity after short-term weight restoration. *Int J Eat Disord*, **89**: 57–68.

Friedman JM (2000) Obesity in the new millennium. *Nature*, **404**: 632–4.

Geliebter A and Hashim SA (2001) Gastric capacity in normal, obese, and bulimic women. *Physiol Behav*, **89**: 743–6.

Geliebter A, Yahav EK, Gluck ME and Hashim SA (2004) Gastric capacity, test meal intake, and appetitive hormones in binge eating disorder. *Physiol Behav*, **89**: 735–40.

Gendall KA, Kaye WH, Altemus M, McConaha CW and La Via MC (1999) Leptin, neuropeptide Y, and peptide YY in long-term recovered eating disorder patients. *Biol Psychiatry*, **89**: 292–9.

Goethals I, Vervaet M, Audenaert K, Van de WC, Ham H, Vandecapelle M *et al.* (2004) Comparison of cortical 5-HT2A receptor binding in bulimia nervosa patients and healthy volunteers. *Am J Psychiatry*, **161**: 1916–18.

Hebebrand J, Blum WF, Barth N, Coners H, Englaro P, Juul A *et al.* (1997) Leptin levels in patients with anorexia nervosa are reduced in the acute stage and elevated upon short-term weight restoration. *Mol Psychiatry*, **2**: 330–4.

Hebebrand J, Exner C, Hebebrand K, Holtkamp C, Casper RC, Remschmidt H *et al.* (2003) Hyperactivity in patients with anorexia nervosa and in semistarved rats: evidence for a pivotal role of hypoleptinemia. *Physiol Behav*, **89**: 25–37.

Heisler LK, Cowley MA, Kishi T, Tecott LH, Fan W, Low MJ *et al.* (2003) Central serotonin and melanocortin pathways regulating energy homeostasis. *Ann N Y Acad Sci*, **994**: 169–74.

Holtkamp K, Hebebrand J, Mika C, Grzella I, Heer M, Heussen N *et al.* (2003a) The effect of therapeutically induced weight gain on plasma leptin levels in patients with anorexia nervosa. *J Psychiatr Res*, **89**: 165–9.

Holtkamp K, Herpertz-Dahlmann B, Mika C, Heer M, Heussen N, Fichter M *et al.* (2003b) Elevated physical activity and low leptin levels co-occur in patients with anorexia nervosa. *J Clin Endocrinol Metab*, **89**: 5169–74.

Holtkamp K, Mika C, Grzella I, Heer M, Pak H, Hebebrand J *et al.* (2003c) Reproductive function during weight gain in anorexia nervosa. Leptin represents a metabolic gate to gonadotropin secretion. *J Neural Transm*, **110**: 427–35.

Holtkamp K, Hebebrand J, Mika C, Heer M, Heussen N and Herpertz-Dahlmann B (2004) High serum leptin levels subsequent to weight gain predict renewed weight loss in patients with anorexia nervosa. *Psychoneuroendocrinology*, **29**: 791–7.

Hotta M, Ohwada R, Katakami H, Shibasaki T, Hizuka N and Takano K (2004) Plasma levels of intact and degraded ghrelin and their responses to glucose infusion in anorexia nervosa. *J Clin Endocrinol Metab*, **89**: 5707–12.

Housova J, Anderlova K, Krizova J, Haluzikova D, Kremen J, Kumstyrova T *et al.* (2005) Serum adiponectin and resistin concentrations in patients with restrictive and binge/purge form of anorexia nervosa and bulimia nervosa. *J Clin Endocrinol Metab*, **90**: 1366–70.

Inui A (2005) Acyl and desacyl ghrelin in anorexia nervosa. *Psychoneuroendocrinology*, **30**: 115.

Iwahashi H, Funahashi T, Kurokawa N, Sayama K, Fukuda E, Okita K *et al.* (2003) Plasma adiponectin levels in women with anorexia nervosa. *Horm Metab Res*, **35**: 537–40.

Jimerson DC and Wolfe BE (2004) Neuropeptides in eating disorders. *CNS Spectr*, **9**: 516–22.

Jimerson DC, Wolfe BE, Metzger ED, Finkelstein DM, Cooper TB and Levine JM (1997) Decreased serotonin function in bulimia nervosa. *Arch Gen Psychiatry*, **54**: 529–34.

Jimerson DC, Mantzoros C, Wolfe BE and Metzger ED (2000) Decreased serum leptin in bulimia nervosa. *J Clin Endocrinol Metab*, **85**: 4511–14.

Kaye WH, Gwirtsman HE, George DT and Ebert MH (1991) Altered serotonin activity in anorexia nervosa after long-term weight restoration. Does elevated cerebrospinal fluid 5-hydroxyindoleacetic acid level correlate with rigid and obsessive behavior? *Arch Gen Psychiatry*, **48**: 556–62.

Kaye WH, Greeno CG, Moss H, Fernstrom J, Fernstrom M, Lilenfeld LR *et al.* (1998) Alterations in serotonin activity and psychiatric symptoms after recovery from bulimia nervosa. *Arch Gen Psychiatry*, **55**: 927–35.

Kaye WH, Gendall KA, Fernstrom MH, Fernstrom JD, McConaha CW and Weltzin TE (2000) Effects of acute tryptophan depletion on mood in bulimia nervosa. *Biol Psychiatry*, **47**: 151–7.

Kaye WH, Frank GK, Meltzer CC, Price JC, McConaha CW, Crossan PJ *et al.* (2001) Altered serotonin 2A receptor activity in women who have recovered from bulimia nervosa. *Am J Psychiatry*, **158**: 1152–5.

***Kaye WH, Barbarich NC, Putnam K, Gendall KA, Fernstrom J, Fernstrom M *et al.* (2003) Anxiolytic effects of acute tryptophan depletion in anorexia nervosa. *Int J Eat Disord*, **33**: 257–67.

This article provides a notable follow-up to work from this laboratory indicating that women who have recovered from anorexia nervosa demonstrate persistent overactivity in CNS serotonergic pathways. In this placebo-controlled study, the authors showed that acute tryptophan depletion, which is thought to decrease CNS serotonin synthesis, resulted in decreased symptoms of anxiety in low-weight patients and in weight-recovered individuals. The authors offer an intriguing speculation that one reason why patients diet may be to reduce a dysphoric mood state.

Kaye WH, Strober M and Jimerson DC (2004) The neurobiology of eating disorders. In: DS Charney and EJ Nestler (eds), *The Neurobiology of Mental Illness*. Oxford University Press, Oxford, pp 1112–28.

Kojima S, Nakahara T, Nagai N, Muranaga T, Tanaka M, Yasuhara D *et al.* (2005) Altered ghrelin and peptide YY responses to meals in bulimia nervosa. *Clin Endocrinol (Oxf)*, **62**: 74–8.

Kratzsch J, Lammert A, Bottner A, Seidel B, Mueller G, Thiery J *et al.* (2002) Circulating soluble leptin receptor and free leptin index during childhood, puberty, and adolescence. *J Clin Endocrinol Metab*, **87**: 4587–94.

Krizova J, Papezova H, Haluzikova D, Parizkova J, Jiskra J, Kotrlikova E *et al.* (2002) Soluble leptin receptor levels in patients with anorexia nervosa. *Endocrinol Res*, **28**: 199–205.

Krsek M, Rosicka M, Papezova H, Krizova J, Kotrlikova E, Haluz'k M *et al.* (2003) Plasma ghrelin levels and malnutrition: a comparison of two etiologies. *Eat Weight Disord*, **8**: 207–11.

Kuikka JT, Tammela L, Karhunen L, Rissanen A, Bergstrom KA, Naukkarinen H *et al.* (2001) Reduced serotonin transporter binding in binge eating women. *Psychopharmacology (Berl)*, **155**: 310–14.

Leidy HJ, Gardner JK, Frye BR, Snook ML, Schuchert MK, Richard EL *et al.* (2004) Circulating ghrelin is sensitive to changes in body weight during a diet and exercise program in normal-weight young women. *J Clin Endocrinol Metab*, **89**: 2659–64.

Lob S, Pickel J, Bidlingmaier M, Schaaf L, Backmund H, Gerlinghoff M *et al.* (2003) Serum leptin monitoring in anorectic patients during refeeding therapy. *Exp Clin Endocrinol Diabetes*, **111**: 278–82.

Mantzoros C, Flier JS, Lesem MD, Brewerton TD and Jimerson DC (1997) Cerebrospinal fluid leptin in anorexia nervosa: correlation with nutritional status and potential role in resistance to weight gain. *J Clin Endocrinol Metab*, **82**: 1845–51.

Miller KK, Grinspoon S, Gleysteen S, Grieco KA, Ciampa J, Breu J *et al.* (2004) Preservation of neuroendocrine control of reproductive function despite severe undernutrition. *J Clin Endocrinol Metab*, **89**: 4434–8.

Misra M, Miller KK, Almazan C, Ramaswamy K, Aggarwal A, Herzog DB *et al.* (2004a) Hormonal and body composition predictors of soluble leptin receptor, leptin, and free leptin index in adolescent girls with anorexia nervosa and controls and relation to insulin sensitivity. *J Clin Endocrinol Metab*, **89**: 3486–95.

Misra M, Miller KK, Herzog DB, Ramaswamy K, Aggarwal A, Almazan C *et al.* (2004b) Growth hormone and ghrelin responses to an oral glucose load in adolescent girls with anorexia nervosa and controls. *J Clin Endocrinol Metab*, **89**: 1605–12.

Monteleone P, Brambilla F, Bortolotti F and Maj M (2000) Serotonergic dysfunction across the eating disorders: relationship to eating behavior, purging behavior, nutritional status and general psychopathology. *Psychol Med*, **30**: 1099–110.

Monteleone P, Fabrazzo M, Tortorella A, Fuschino A and Maj M (2002) Opposite modifications in circulating leptin and soluble leptin receptor across the eating disorder spectrum. *Mol Psychiatry*, **7**: 641–6.

Monteleone P, Fabrazzo M, Martiadis V, Fuschino A, Serritella C, Milici N *et al.* (2003a) Opposite changes in circulating adiponectin in women with bulimia nervosa or binge eating disorder. *J Clin Endocrinol Metab*, **88**: 5387–91.

***Monteleone P, Martiadis V, Fabrazzo M, Serritella C and Maj M (2003b) Ghrelin and leptin responses to food ingestion in bulimia nervosa: implications for binge-eating and compensatory behaviors. *Psychol Med*, **33**: 1387–94.

This well-designed study showed that the postprandial suppression of plasma levels of ghrelin which is observed in healthy volunteers is significantly blunted in patients with bulimia nervosa. This finding is consistent with earlier test-meal studies showing blunted ratings of satiety following a test-meal in patients with this disorder. Also of interest are the similar findings reported for binge-eating disorder by Geliebter *et al.* (2004).

Monteleone P, DiLieto A, Castaldo E and Maj M (2004) Leptin functioning in eating disorders. *CNS Spectr*, **9**: 523–9.

Monteleone P, Fabrazzo M, Tortorella A, Martiadis V, Serritella C and Maj M (2005) Circulating ghrelin is decreased in non-obese and obese women with binge eating disorder as well as in obese non-binge eating women, but not in patients with bulimia nervosa. *Psychoneuroendocrinology*, **30**: 243–50.

Nakai Y, Hosoda H, Nin K, Ooya C, Hayashi H, Akamizu T *et al.* (2003) Plasma levels of active form of ghrelin during oral glucose tolerance test in patients with anorexia nervosa. *Eur J Endocrinol*, **149**: R1–R3.

Nakazato M, Hashimoto K, Shiina A, Koizumi H, Mitsumoti M, Imai M *et al.* (2004) No changes in serum ghrelin levels in female patients with bulimia nervosa. *Prog Neuropsychopharmacol Biol Psychiatry*, **28**: 1181–4.

Neary NM, Small CJ and Bloom SR (2003) Gut and mind. *Gut*, **52**: 918–21.

Nedvídková J, Krykorkova I, Barták V, Papezová H, Gold PW, Alesci S *et al.* (2003) Loss of meal-induced decrease in plasma ghrelin levels in patients with anorexia nervosa. *J Clin Endocrinol Metab*, **88**: 1678–82.

O'Dwyer AM, Lucey JV and Russell GF (1996) Serotonin activity in anorexia nervosa after long-term weight restoration: response to D-fenfluramine challenge. *Psychol Med*, **26**: 353–9.

Otto B, Cuntz U, Fruehauf E, Wawarta R, Folwaczny C, Riepl RL *et al.* (2001) Weight gain decreases elevated plasma ghrelin concentrations of patients with anorexia nervosa. *Eur J Endocrinol*, **145**: 669–73.

Otto B, Tschop M and Cuntz U (2004) Letter to the Editor: Similar fasting ghrelin levels in binge eating/purging anorexia nervosa and restrictive anorexia nervosa. *Psychoneuroendocrinology*, **29**: 692–3.

Pannacciulli N, Vettor R, Milan G, Granzotto M, Catucci A, Federspil G *et al.* (2003) Anorexia nervosa is characterized by increased adiponectin plasma levels and reduced nonoxidative glucose metabolism. *J Clin Endocrinol Metab*, **88**: 1748–52.

Popovic V, Djurovic M, Cetkovic A, Vojvodic D, Pekic S, Spremovic S *et al.* (2004) Inhibin B: a potential marker of gonadal activity in patients with anorexia nervosa during weight recovery. *J Clin Endocrinol Metab*, **89**: 1838–43.

Ramacciotti CE, Coli E, Paoli R, Marazziti D and Dell'Osso L (2003) Serotonergic activity measured by platelet [3H]paroxetine binding in patients with eating disorders. *Psychiatry Res*, **118**: 33–8.

Rigamonti AE, Pincelli AI, Corra B, Viarengo R, Bonomo SM, Galimberti D *et al.* (2002) Plasma ghrelin concentrations in elderly subjects: comparison with anorexic and obese patients. *J Endocrinol*, **175**: R1–R5.

Shiiya T, Nakazato M, Mizuta M, Date Y, Mondal MS, Tanaka M *et al.* (2002) Plasma ghrelin levels in lean and obese humans and the effect of glucose on ghrelin secretion. *J Clin Endocrinol Metab*, **87**: 240–4.

Smith KA, Fairburn CG and Cowen PJ (1999) Symptomatic relapse in bulimia nervosa following acute tryptophan depletion. *Arch Gen Psychiatry*, **56**: 171–6.

Soriano-Guillén L, Barrios V, Campos-Barros A and Argente J (2004) Ghrelin levels in obesity and anorexia nervosa: effect of weight reduction or recuperation. *J Pediatr*, **144**: 36–42.

Steiger H (2004) Eating disorders and the serotonin connection: state, trait and developmental effects. *J Psychiatry Neurosci*, **29**: 20–9.

Steiger H, Gauvin L, Israel M, Koerner N, Ng Ying Kin NM, Paris J *et al.* (2001a) Association of serotonin and cortisol indices with childhood abuse in bulimia nervosa. *Arch Gen Psychiatry*, **58**: 837–43.

Steiger H, Koerner N, Engelberg MJ, Israel M, Ng Ying Kin NM and Young SN (2001b) Self-destructiveness and serotonin function in bulimia nervosa. *Psychiatry Res*, **103**: 15–26.

***Steiger H, Israel M, Gauvin L, Ng Ying Kin NM and Young SN (2003) Implications of compulsive and impulsive traits for serotonin status in women with bulimia nervosa. *Psychiatry Res*, **120**: 219–29.

A series of neuroendocrine and platelet studies from this laboratory has shown that bulimia nervosa appears to be associated with a decrement in serotonin function, extending similar findings in earlier reports from other investigators. Taken in conjunction with previous work from this laboratory, this study suggests that patients with the greatest reduction in serotonergic measures are the most likely to demonstrate impulsive behavioral characteristics.

Steiger H, Gauvin L, Israel M, Kin NM, Young SN and Roussin J (2004) Serotonin function, personality-trait variations, and childhood abuse in women with bulimia-spectrum eating disorders. *J Clin Psychiatry*, **65**: 830–7.

Stock S, Leichner P, Wong AC, Ghatei MA, Kieffer TJ, Bloom SR *et al.* (2005) Ghrelin, peptide YY, glucose-dependent insulinotropic polypeptide and hunger responses to a mixed meal in anorexic, obese and control female adolescents. *J Clin Endocrinol Metab*, **90**: 2161–8.

Tagami T, Satoh N, Usui T, Yamada K, Shimatsu A and Kuzuya H (2004) Adiponectin in anorexia nervosa and bulimia nervosa. *J Clin Endocrinol Metab*, **89**: 1833–7.

Tammela LI, Rissanen A, Kuikka JT, Karhunen LJ, Bergstrom KA, Repo-Tiihonen E *et al.* (2003) Treatment improves serotonin transporter binding and reduces binge eating. *Psychopharmacology*, **170**: 89–93.

Tanaka M, Naruo T, Muranaga T, Yasuhara D, Shiiya T, Nakazato M *et al.* (2002) Increased fasting plasma ghrelin levels in patients with bulimia nervosa. *Eur J Endocrinol*, **146**: R1–R3.

Tanaka M, Naruo T, Nagai N, Kuroki N, Shiiya T, Nakazato M *et al.* (2003a) Habitual binge/purge behavior influences circulating ghrelin levels in eating disorders. *J Psychiatr Res*, **37**: 17–22.

Tanaka M, Naruo T, Yasuhara D, Tatebe Y, Nagai N, Shiiya T *et al.* (2003b) Fasting plasma ghrelin levels in subtypes of anorexia nervosa. *Psychoneuroendocrinology*, **28**: 829–35.

Tanaka M, Tatebe Y, Nakahara T, Yasuhara D, Sagiyama K, Muranaga T *et al.* (2003c) Eating pattern and the effect of oral glucose on ghrelin and insulin secretion in patients with anorexia nervosa. *Clin Endocrinol*, **59**: 574–9.

Tanaka M, Nakahara T, Kojima S, Nakano T, Muranaga T, Nagai N *et al.* (2004) Effect of nutritional rehabilitation on circulating ghrelin and growth hormone levels in patients with anorexia nervosa. *Regul Pept*, **122**: 163–8.

Tauscher J, Pirker W, Willeit M, de Zwaan M, Bailer U, Neumeister A *et al.* (2001) [^{123}I] b-CIT and single photon emission computed tomography reveal reduced brain serotonin transporter availability in bulimia nervosa. *Biol Psychiatry*, **49**: 326–32.

Tiihonen J, Keski-Rahkonen A, Lopponen M, Muhonen M, Kajander J, Allonen T *et al.* (2004) Brain serotonin 1A receptor binding in bulimia nervosa. *Biol Psychiatry*, **55**: 871–3.

Tolle V, Kadem M, Bluet-Pajot MT, Frere D, Foulon C, Bossu C *et al.* (2003) Balance in ghrelin and leptin plasma levels in anorexia nervosa patients and constitutionally thin women. *J Clin Endocrinol Metab*, **88**: 109–16.

Tomasik PJ, Sztefko K and Starzyk J (2004) Cholecystokinin, glucose dependent insulino-tropic peptide and glucagon-like peptide 1 secretion in children with anorexia nervosa and simple obesity. *J Pediatr Endocrinol Metab*, **17**: 1623–31.

Walsh BT, Zimmerli E, Devlin MJ, Guss J and Kissileff HR (2003) A disturbance of gastric function in bulimia nervosa. *Biol Psychiatry*, **54**: 929–33.

Ward A, Brown N, Lightman S, Campbell IC and Treasure J (1998) Neuroendocrine, appetitive and behavioral responses to d-fenfluramine in women recovered from anorexia nervosa. *Br J Psychiatry*, **172**: 351–8.

Wolfe BE, Metzger E and Jimerson DC (1997) Research update on serotonin function in bulimia nervosa and anorexia nervosa. *Psychopharmacol Bull*, **33**: 345–54.

Wolfe BE, Metzger ED, Levine JM, Finkelstein DM, Cooper TB and Jimerson DC (2000) Serotonin function following remission from bulimia nervosa. *Neuropsychopharmacology*, **22**: 257–63.

Wolfe BE, Jimerson DC, Orlova C and Mantzoros CS (2004) Effect of dieting on plasma leptin, soluble leptin receptor, adiponectin and resistin levels in healthy volunteers. *Clin Endocrinol*, **61**: 332–8.

Wren AM, Seal LJ, Cohen MA, Brynes AE, Frost GS, Murphy KG *et al.* (2001) Ghrelin enhances appetite and increases food intake in humans. *J Clin Endocrinol Metab*, **86**: 5992–5.

Zastrow O, Seidel B, Kiess W, Thiery J, Keller E, Bottner A *et al.* (2003) The soluble leptin receptor is crucial for leptin action: evidence from clinical and experimental data. *Int J Obes Relat Metab Disord*, **27**: 1472–8.

Zigman JM and Elmquist JK (2003) Minireview: From anorexia to obesity–the yin and yang of body weight control. *Endocrinology*, **144**: 3749–56.

2

Genetics of eating disorders

Suzanne E Mazzeo, Margarita CT Slof-Op't Landt,
Eric F van Furth and Cynthia M Bulik

Abstract

Objectives of review. The aim of this paper is to review the major genetic studies of eating disorders (EDs) conducted within the last two years.
Summary of recent findings. Twin studies have highlighted the importance of both genetic and environmental factors in ED etiology. In addition, these studies have indicated that some specific ED-related attitudes are significantly associated with environmental factors. These findings have important implications for prevention. In addition, linkage and association studies have further specified several important candidate genes and their relevance to ED behavior and attitudes.
Future directions. The studies published over the last two years highlight the importance of measuring EDs at the symptom level, as risk factors appear to be somewhat symptom specific. In addition, studies using samples that include various age cohorts have indicated that there are distinct genetic and environmental risk factors for EDs within different age groups. Thus, future studies should continue to use members of different cohorts in their samples. In addition, longitudinal designs will continue to be of value.

Introduction

The past decade has witnessed a virtual explosion of research on the genetic epidemiology and molecular genetics of eating disorders (EDs). Following decades of EDs being considered to be primarily environmentally determined, it is now generally accepted that EDs aggregate in families, that a considerable proportion of familial aggregation is due to genetic factors, and that efforts to identify genes or alleles that confer risk of EDs are rational and appropriate. Studies published in the past two years have continued to shed light on patterns of familial transmission of various EDs and eating disorder-related behaviors and have revealed several genes and gene pathways that may be implicated in ED risk.

Literature review

Family and twin studies

Family and twin studies have been extremely influential in identifying genetic and environmental contributions to ED etiology, and their findings have supported efforts to identify loci that influence risk for these disorders and associated traits. In the following paragraphs we review studies that have used twin or family methodology to investigate specific ED features.

Binge eating and binge-eating disorder

Binge eating (BE) as a symptom and binge-eating disorder (BED) as a syndrome have received significant attention in the last few years, as awareness has increased regarding both the prevalence of this behavior and its relevance to obesity. Three recent studies have examined the familial aggregation and heritability of BE. In the first (Hudson *et al.* 2004), family members of overweight or obese individuals with and without BED were assessed. Individuals who had a family member with BED were more than twice as likely to have BED themselves, compared to those with an overweight or obese relative without BED.

Bulik and colleagues (Bulik *et al.* 2003a) examined genetic and environmental contributions to BE and obesity in a US (Virginia) population-based twin sample. They found that obesity and BE shared a significant, although moderate, proportion of genetic variance (r_g=.34), suggesting that both traits are influenced by some of the same genetic factors. Moreover, obesity appeared to be highly heritable (a^2=.86), whereas BE was moderately heritable (a^2=.49). BE was also strongly associated with unique environmental factors (e^2=.51). Based on these findings, the investigators concluded that obesity does not cause BE, nor does BE cause obesity. Rather, both appear to be heritable, and to be caused by some, but not all, of the same genetic factors.

A third study, conducted by Reichborn-Kjennerud and colleagues (Reichborn-Kjennerud *et al.* 2003), investigated gender differences in BE using the population-based Norwegian twin registry. BE was moderately heritable for both men and women (a^2=.51); common environmental factors did not significantly contribute to BE. Moreover, the proportion of genetic variance in BE shared between men and women was estimated at 0.57 (95% CI 0.07–1.00), indicating that the majority of genetic risk factors for BE are shared across genders. Gender-specific factors could not, however, be ruled out entirely.

Eating and weight-related behaviors and attitudes

Three recent twin studies examined the influence of genetic and environmental factors on ED-related attitudes and behaviors. The first of these (Klump *et al.* 2003) examined Minnesota Eating Disorders Inventory (M-EDI) scores in prepubertal and postpubertal 11-year-old twin girls. These twins were also compared to a 17-year-old twin cohort. All participants were part of the Minnesota Twin Family Study. Previous research has found that the influence of genetic factors on ED symptomatology increases significantly during the adolescent years (Klump *et al.* 2000). Thus, in the current study, the authors hypothesized that genetic factors would be more strongly associated with M-EDI scores in postpubertal 11-year-old girls, compared to the preubertal subsample; this hypothesis was supported. Specifically, in prepubertal twins, no significant influence of additive genetic factors was evident, yet common environmental factors were important (c^2=.53). In contrast, in both postpubertal 11-year-old and 17-year-old girls, genetic effects were significant (a^2=.54 for both groups), and shared environment was not associated with M-EDI scores. These results further support the idea that genes relevant to EDs are activated during puberty in young women.

Gender differences in genetic and environmental contributions to Eating Disorder Inventory (EDI) Body Dissatisfaction (BD) and Drive for Thinness (DT) scores were examined in the population-based FinnTwin16 project (Keski-Rahkonen *et al.* 2005). In the best-fitting model, no additive genetic contributions to DT or BD were detected in males. Rather, common environmental or dominance factors accounted for most of the variance in men's scores on DT (c^2/d^2=.86, CI 84.4–88.0), and BD (c^2/d^2=.86, CI 84.4–88.0). In contrast, DT and BD heritability estimates for female twins were relatively strong (i.e. a^2_{DFT}=.51, CI 43.7–57.5; a^2_{BD}=.59, CI 53.2–64.7), and environmental factors did not contribute to the variance of these traits. Taken together, these results suggest that the heritability patterns of these ED-related attitudes are highly gender specific. However, it should be noted that the EDI, particularly the BD subscale, focuses on core areas of female body and weight dissatisfaction (e.g. hips, buttocks). Thus, the EDI is not an ideal measure of male body shape-related attitudes, as domains of importance such as muscularity and stature are ignored.

Gender differences were also investigated in a recent study conducted with Norwegian Twin Panel data by Reichborn-Kjennerud *et al.* (2004). Specifically, these researchers evaluated the contribution of genetic and environmental factors to the tendency to place undue importance on weight as an indicator of self-evaluation. The best-fitting model did not reveal any genetic contribution to this trait in men or women. Rather, specific and shared environmental factors accounted for most of the variance. Moreover, gender differences in the influence of these factors were not detected. It is noteworthy that common environmental factors were associated with this trait (c^2=.31), as many ED-related behaviors have been found to be largely accounted for by additive genetic factors (e.g. Reichborn-Kjennerud *et al.* 2003). However, results of this study are consistent with those of Wade and colleagues (Wade *et al.* 1998) who found that ED Examination Weight Concern scale scores (which also assess the undue influence of bodyweight on self-concept) were best accounted for by a combination of shared and specific environmental factors. In sum, these findings suggest that although genetic factors play a substantial role in the development of several ED symptoms, environmental factors also make important contributions to certain features of the ED phenotype. Moreover, these results further highlight the importance of evaluating symptom-level (rather than diagnosis-level) manifestations of eating pathology, as different symptoms (e.g. body dissatisfaction, purging) may have distinct patterns of familial resemblance.

The relevance of both environmental and genetic factors to the etiology of EDs was also noted in a recent investigation of genetic and environmental influences on female twins' Eating Inventory (also known as the Three-Factor Eating Questionnaire, TFEQ) scores (Neale *et al.* 2003). Specifically, these authors found that scores on the Restraint subscale were associated with shared (c^2=.31, CI .04–.42) and specific (e^2=.69, CI .58–.80) environmental factors. Additive genetic effects did not contribute to Restraint scores. Similar results were obtained for the Hunger subscale. In contrast, Disinhibition scores (which indicate one's tendency to eat or overeat in response to contextual cues) were significantly influenced by additive genetic factors (a^2=.45, CI .32–.57); common environment did not contribute to variance in scores on this subscale. These results suggest that dieting, as measured by the Restraint subscale, is a learned behavior. This may have important implications for ED prevention, as will be discussed in a subsequent section.

Eating disorders and psychiatric comorbidities

Two recent studies have examined associations between EDs and psychiatric comorbidities. First, Grigoroiu-Serbanescu and colleagues (Grigoroiu-Serbanescu *et al.* 2003) conducted a longitudinal investigation of psychopathology in relatives of individuals with Anorexia Nervosa-Restricting Subtype (AN-R), and found that female relatives were more likely than controls to meet criteria for an anxiety disorder or major depression.

The association among these disorders was also supported in a study conducted by Silberg and Bulik (in press), which examined the influence of genetic and environmental factors on EDs, anxiety disorders, and depression in 8–13- and 14–17-year-old twin girls. They found that early EDs were associated with a unique additive genetic effect. Yet, early EDs were further associated with a common environmental effect that was also related to depression. In contrast, later EDs were associated with a genetic factor that was also related to depression and anxiety disorders. In addition, later EDs were associated with a common environmental factor that was also related to both early and later separation anxiety disorder. This study is consistent with Klump *et al.*'s (2003) finding that genetic and environmental factors differentially contributed to pre- and post-pubertal EDs. However, unlike Klump and colleagues, Silberg and Bulik identified a significant influence of additive genetic factors on prepubertal EDs. They propose that this finding may be due to either the greater power of their study or their use of child-specific measures. Although additional studies are needed to clarify these discrepancies, these findings highlight the importance of assessing EDs and associated comorbidities across the lifespan.

Molecular genetic studies

The number of studies focusing on the role of genetics in the etiology of EDs has increased exponentially in recent years. Molecular genetic investigations of EDs use two methodologies: linkage and association analyses (Slagboom and Meulenbelt 2002). In linkage analysis, variation in the paternal and maternal contribution to the various genomes of the offspring is used to localize disease genes or genes that influence a trait (Slagboom and Meulenbelt 2002). For this approach, a large sample of multiplex pedigrees or extreme sibling pairs (pairs that are either concordant for high or low values, or extremely discordant for a certain trait) is required (Kruglyak *et al.* 1996).

In a genetic association study, cases that display a trait of interest are compared to controls who do not display the trait. One or several candidate genes are genotyped in all individuals, and the allele and genotype frequencies are compared in cases versus controls (Slagboom and Meulenbelt 2002). A disadvantage of this design is the risk of yielding false-positive results, due to population stratification. However, in addition to case–control designs, an association study can also be performed in family trios, by using a Transmission Disequilibrium Test (TDT). In general, a family trio is composed of an affected individual and both biological parents. In the TDT approach, the transmission versus non-transmission of marker alleles to affected offspring is compared (Schulze and McMahon 2002). The major advantage of this method is that it eliminates population stratification effects completely. The following sections briefly review the major linkage and association studies that have been conducted in the area of EDs within the last two years.

Linkage studies

Bulik *et al.* (2003b) conducted a genome-wide linkage analysis in 316 families in which at least two biological relatives were affected with BN. Significant linkage was identified on chromosome 10, and suggestive linkage was evident on chromosome 14. Next, because previous research has indicated that vomiting is both among the most reliably measured BN-related behaviors and is highly heritable (Sullivan *et al.* 1998), the investigators conducted the linkage analysis within a subset of families in which at least two affected individuals reported self-induced vomiting, thereby increasing the homogeneity of the sample. Within this subsample, significant linkage was found on chromosome 10, and the linkage on chromosome 14 remained suggestive.

This same group followed up on previous findings from their linkage studies of AN (which found evidence of linkage on chromosome 1) (Devlin *et al.* 2002; Grice *et al.* 2002), by identifying neurobiological candidate genes located in this linkage region and conducting both linkage and association analyses using these candidate genes (Bergen *et al.* 2003). The two candidate genes selected for analyses were the serotonin 1D receptor (HTR1D) and the opioid delta receptor (OPRD1), both located at chr1p36.3-34.3. These candidate genes were evaluated for sequence variation and for linkage and association of this sequence variation to AN in family and case–control data sets. Resequencing of the HTR1D locus and a portion of the OPRD1 locus identified novel single nucleotide polymorphisms (SNPs) and confirmed existing SNPs. Genotype assay development and genotyping of nine SNPs (four at HTR1D and five at OPRD1) was performed on 191 unrelated individuals fulfilling DSM-IV criteria (w/o amenorrhea criterion) for AN, 442 relatives of AN probands and 98 psychiatrically screened controls. Linkage analysis of these candidate gene SNPs with 33 microsatellite markers in families including relative pairs concordantly affected with AN-R ($n=37$) substantially increased the evidence for linkage of this region to AN-R to a nonparametric linkage (NPL) score of 3.91. Statistically significant genotypic, allelic and haplotypic association to AN in the case–control design was observed at HTR1D and OPRD1 with maximum effect sizes for individual SNPs of 2.63 (95% CI 1.21–5.75) for HTR1D and 1.61 (95% CI 1.11–2.44) for OPRD1. Using genotype data on parents and AN probands, three SNPs at HTR1D were found to exhibit significant transmission disequilibrium ($p<0.05$). The combined statistical genetic evidence suggests that HTR1D and OPRD1 or linked genes may be involved in the etiology of AN. In sum, this group of investigators have focused in on two promising regions of the genome for AN and BN and are beginning to explore genes in those regions that, based on both position and function, may confer risk to EDs.

Genetic association studies

In addition to linkage studies, researchers have focused their attention on specific candidate genes for EDs. In particular, we identified six articles that examined the association between brain-derived neurotropic factor (BDNF) and EDs. Several other articles examined the relevance of serotonin transporter and receptor genes to EDs. Finally, a few studies investigated other promising candidates, including the monamine oxidase A (MAO-A), cannabinoid receptor (CNR1), and potassium channel (KCNN3) genes. We review studies in each of these areas in the following paragraphs.

BDNF and EDs

Several authors have suggested that polymorphisms in the BDNF gene (located on chromosome 11) may play a role in the pathophysiology of EDs (Ribasés *et al.*

2003, 2004, 2005; Koizumi *et al.* 2004; Friedel *et al.* 2005). BDNF is associated with regulation of bodyweight and appetite in animal models (see Friedel *et al.* 2005 for a review). In addition, a recent study found that BDNF levels of women with EDs were lower than those of controls (Nakazato *et al.* 2003). Moreover, BDNF levels were lower among patients with AN, compared to those with BN, and BDNF was positively associated with BMI in the total sample. However, it is unclear from this non-genetic, correlational study whether EDs were a cause or consequence of reduced BDNF levels. Variants of the BDNF gene have also been found to be associated with obsessive-compulsive disorder (Hall *et al.* 2003), a diagnosis that shares some features of AN.

Recent investigations into the association between polymorphisms of the BDNF gene and EDs have yielded somewhat conflicting, yet generally promising, results. Ribasés and colleagues (Ribasés *et al.* 2003) used a case–control design and found that AN-R was significantly associated with the BDNF Met66 variant. In addition, this variant was significantly associated with minimum BMI. However, the Met66 variant was not associated with either of the other ED subtypes assessed, or with the age of onset of weight loss. Based on these results, the authors suggest that different ED subtypes may have distinct susceptibility factors.

In a subsequent study (Ribasés *et al.* 2005), this group further examined the BDNF-ED association in a larger sample consisting of individuals with EDs recruited from eight European countries, using a TDT approach. Results supported these authors' previous findings (Ribasés *et al.* 2003) regarding the association between the Met66 variant and AN-R. However, they also found that the -270C/T polymorphism was associated with AN-R and minimum BMI. This association was non-significant in their earlier study. Neither polymorphism identified in the second study was associated with either BN or anorexia nervosa/binge eating/purging subtype (AN-BP).

A third study by the same group (Ribasés *et al.* 2004) used a case–control design and included participants from five European countries. Findings suggested that patients with AN-R, AN-BP and BN were all more likely to be carriers of the Met66 variant. BN was also associated with the -270C>T SNP in two of the samples. Late age of weight loss onset was also associated with -270C>T.

An association between BDNF polymorphisms and EDs was also observed by Koizumi and colleagues (Koizumi *et al.* 2004) who found that, compared to controls, patients were more likely to have the BDNF 196G/A (val66met) polymorphism (G/A heterogeneity). Specifically, patients with AN-R and purging BN were more likely than controls to manifest G/A heterogeneity. It is unclear why this polymorphism would be associated with two relatively distinct forms of ED pathology (AN-R and BN-P), and not associated with AN-BP or BN-NP. However, these results should be regarded with some caution, as sample sizes were somewhat small when EDs were broken down into specific subtypes (i.e. $n=36$ AN-R, $n=36$ AN-BP, $n=101$ BN-P, and $n=17$ BN-NP). Thus, failure to identify associations between each ED subtype and these BDNF polymorphisms may be due to inadequate statistical power.

However, in a study conducted by Friedel *et al.* (2005), no associations were found between the Met66 variant and EDs. Unlike the previous studies, Friedel and colleagues included extremely obese children and adolescents, healthy underweight students, and normal weight controls, as well as patients with EDs. The authors do not note how many of the patients with AN had the AN-R or AN-BP subtype. It is possible that too few patients with AN-R were included in Friedel *et al.*'s study to detect an association between this ED subtype and Met66.

In sum, although research examining the association between BDNF polymorphisms and EDs is at an early stage, there have been several investigations conducted in this area within the last two years, and results have been relatively promising. In particular, the Met66 variant appears to be associated with AN-R. Nonetheless, additional research is needed to determine the relevance of this and other BDNF variants to specific ED subtypes. Further, all of the studies published within the last two years, with the exception of Koizumi *et al.* (2004), were conducted in predominantly Caucasian and European samples. Thus, additional research is needed to investigation these relationships across populations.

In addition, as Ribasés *et al.* (2003) caution, the observed association between Met66 and AN-R may be attributable to an as-yet-unobserved association between Met66 and another candidate gene in linkage disequilibrium with it. For example, higher levels of BDNF are also associated with higher extracellular serotonin levels (*see* Ribasés *et al.* 2003). Thus, other important candidates for the EDs include the serotonin transporter and receptor genes. Several recent studies have also focused attention on their contribution to eating pathology.

Genes regulating serotonin

Previous studies have suggested that serotonin (5-HT) may play an important role in the pathophysiology of EDs, particularly AN (Kaye *et al.* 1991, 2001). The serotonin pathway is involved in the regulation of appetite and eating behavior. Individuals who have recovered from AN have persistent 5-HT disturbances (Kaye *et al.* 1991). In addition, selective serotonin reuptake inhibitors (SSRIs) are a useful component of ED treatment (e.g. Kaye *et al.* 2001). These results suggest that hyperserotonergic activity might be a trait marker for EDs. Moreover, serotonin also appears to be associated with some of the psychopathological features of EDs, such as perfectionism, rigidity and obsessionality (Hinney *et al.* 2000). Based on these findings, the 5-HT transporter and receptor genes have been the focus of several studies published within the last two years.

Serotonin transporter (5-HTTLPR/SLC6A4)

A functional polymorphism has been identified in the promoter region of the serotonin transporter gene. This common polymorphism consists of repeats with two major alleles: a long allele (insertion of 16 repeat elements) and a short allele (deletion of 44 base pairs). The short allele (S) is associated with reduced transcriptional efficiency (Heils *et al.* 1996).

Matsushita and colleagues (Matsushita *et al.* 2004) investigated the association between 5-HTTLPR and eating pathology in a case–control study of Japanese women. They found that the S/S genotype and S allele of the 5-HTTLPR gene occurred more frequently in individuals with AN than controls; this increased S allele frequency was evident in both AN subtypes. Moreover, the S allele was most common among those diagnosed with persistent AN (defined as AN lasting at least three years), suggesting that it may be associated with a chronic illness course. No differences in S allele frequencies were found between individuals with BN and controls. These results are consistent with prior investigations, which also found associations among the S allele, S/S genotype and AN (e.g. Di Bella *et al*. 2000). However, Matsushita *et al*. did not replicate the finding of the one previous study to investigate BN and 5-HTTPLR, which found a positive association (Di Bella *et al*. 2000). This inconsistency may be attributable to the fact that Matsushita *et al*. had a larger sample, or to the fact that the S allele occurs more frequently within the Japanese population. Thus, the authors encourage further replication of their findings in diverse populations.

Stieger and colleagues (Stieger *et al*. 2005) used a somewhat different approach, and examined factors associated with 5-HTTPLR within a sample composed exclusively of women (*n*=59) with 'binge-purge syndromes' (which included individuals with BN, eating disorder not otherwise specified (EDNOS) and AN-BP). They found that the S allele was not associated with ED symptoms, including bingeing or vomiting frequency, body dissatisfaction, eating attitudes, or BMI. However, the S allele was associated with borderline personality disorder and related symptoms (including impulsivity, affective instability and insecure attachment). In addition, individuals with the S allele had a significantly lower density of paroxetine binding sites, suggesting that they might not respond as well to traditional SSRIs. Further, the authors note that results regarding paroxetine binding may be due to an interaction of environmental and genetic factors, as animal studies have found that chronic food restriction is associated with 5-HT dysregulation. Thus, perhaps the chronic dieting typical of patients with BN might have triggered the expression of this genetic polymorphism. Future studies are needed to clarify these potential associations. Nonetheless, Stieger *et al*.'s work highlights the importance of both measuring specific traits associated with EDs, and of considering the influence of potential gene–environment interactions that can suggest appropriate targets for intervention.

Epistasis, or the interaction between the SLC6A4 functional polymorphism and a polymorphism of the norepinephrine transporter gene (NET), was also recently investigated in an Australian sample (Urwin *et al*. 2003a) using a TDT approach. Both 5-HTTLPR and NET were associated with AN in prior studies. Consequently, Urwin and colleagues hypothesized that AN might be attributable to the interactive effect of these genes. However, they did not find any evidence of epistasis, nor was there any association between a functional polymorphism in SLC6A4 and AN. These results regarding the lack of association between SLC6A4 and AN are similar to those obtained in two earlier studies (Hinney *et al*. 1997; Sundaramurthy *et al*. 2000). Another recent investigation (Lauzurica *et al*. 2003) also failed to identify differences between patients with BN and controls in frequencies of either the 5-HTTLPR or the variable number of tandem repeat (VNTR) polymorphisms. However, these authors did find that, compared to controls, individuals with BN manifested a higher frequency of the S/S genotype in combination with the 10/12 genotype of a VNTR located at intron 2 of the SLC6A4 gene.

Another study conducted by Urwin and colleagues (Urwin *et al.* 2003b) investigated the potential interaction between the SLC6A4 polymorphism and a polymorphism of the monoamine oxidase A gene. They found that individuals with the MAOA-L allele who were also NETpPR-L4 heterozygotes were twice as likely to have AN-R. Based on these results, the authors concluded that the noradrenergic system, as well as serotonin, is important in the pathophysiology of AN.

Serotonin receptors

Several recent studies have focused on the G-1438A polymorphism in the promoter region of the HTR2A receptor gene. Ricca and colleagues (Ricca *et al.* 2004) investigated this relationship in a case–control study and found that women with EDs were more likely to have an A allele. Moreover, women with AN-R and BN were more likely than controls to have both the A allele and AA genotypes. These investigators also examined the association of Eating Disorder Examination (EDE) scores with G-1438A and found that individuals with the AA genotype had the highest total scores, as well as higher scores on the Weight and Shape Concern subscales. However, a limitation of this study is that the sample of patients with EDs (as well as the subsamples of individuals with AN-BP and BN) deviated from Hardy-Weinberg equilibrium. Nonetheless, this investigation highlights the importance of using both diagnostic criteria as well as continuous measures of ED symptomatology in molecular genetic research.

The association between the G-1438A polymorphism and BN was investigated using a case–control design (Fuentes *et al.* 2004). Results indicated that there was no association between this polymorphism and BN in either the total sample or in subsamples of individuals with and without prior AN diagnoses.

The relevance of the Cys-23-Ser polymorphism, located at the HTR2C receptor gene, to AN was also recently investigated (Hu *et al.* 2003). The frequency of the Ser-23-Ser genotype and the Ser-23 allele was higher among women with AN, compared to controls. Moreover, Ser-23 was associated with minimum BMI. In addition, a TDT analysis in 47 AN trios identified a preferential transmission of the Ser-23 allele. However, only 10 trios were informative for transmission. Thus, although these results are promising, additional studies are needed to confirm involvement of the HTR2C gene in AN.

Finally, Bergen *et al.* (2003) conducted an association study focusing on candidate genes positioned under an observed linkage peak on chromosome 1, one of which was HTR1D. In a case–control design, an association was reported for the C1080T polymorphism and AN. These investigators also performed a TDT analysis which revealed transmission disequilibrium for the A2190G, T-628C and T-1123C polymorphisms, but not for the C1080T polymorphism. Due to the low frequency of the 1080C allele (0.11), only 22 families were informative for this transmission, which might explain why the reported association was not confirmed in the TDT.

Other candidate genes

Gabrovsek and colleagues (Gabrovsek *et al.* 2004) attempted to replicate the work of Frisch *et al.* (2001), who found that the val158Met polymorphism of the catechol-O-methyltransferase gene (COMT) gene was associated with AN. This association was not identified in Gabrovsek *et al.*'s combined family trio and case–control study of individuals from six European countries. Given that these authors used two methodological approaches (case–control and family trio), and their study was sufficiently powered, they concluded that it is unlikely that COMT is associated with AN.

The association between the KCNN3 gene, located on chromosome 1, and AN has also recently been investigated (Koronyo-Hamaoui *et al.* 2004). Patients with AN were more likely than controls to manifest longer CAG repeats of the KCNN3 gene. Interestingly, individuals with AN who manifested the CAG repeat polymorphism were more likely than those without the polymorphism to have comorbid obsessive compulsive disorder (OCD). Based on these findings, the authors recommend that this study be replicated in a larger sample of patients with AN and OCD.

AN was also found to be associated with a polymorphism in the cannabinoid receptor (CNR1) gene in a study using a TDT approach (Siegfried *et al.* 2004). Specifically, AN-BP was associated with the 13-repeat allele of the CNR1 gene, whereas AN-R was associated with the 14-repeat allele. However, the authors note that this study should be replicated as their sample size was relatively small (*n*=52 families).

The relevance of the estrogen receptor β gene (located on chromosome 14) to BN and EDNOS was investigated in a case–control study conducted by Nilsson and colleagues (Nilsson *et al.* 2004). They found that two common polymorphisms in this gene were associated with both ED subtypes assessed.

Shinohara *et al.* (2004) examined the association between a polymorphism in the dopamine transporter gene (DAT1) and binge eating. Patients with EDs (either AN-BP or BN) were more likely to manifest the short allele of the DAT1 gene than controls.

Finally, two recent studies examined the role of melanocortin 4 receptor (MC4R) gene mutations in binge eating. Branson *et al.* (2003) used a case–control design with a sample of 469 severely obese men and women (and 25 non-obese, non-dieting controls). They found that 24 of the obese individuals and one control individual manifested MC4R mutations. Moreover, binge eating was significantly more common among obese individuals with the mutation, compared to obese and control individuals without it. Based on these results, the authors conclude that MC4R is an important candidate gene for binge eating. However, this conclusion should be considered somewhat tentative, as their sample of controls was small. Moreover, 14.5% of obese individuals without the mutation also reported binge eating. A second study investigating MC4R variants and binge eating was recently conducted by Hebebrand and colleagues (Hebebrand *et al.* 2004). These authors identified 43 carriers of potentially functionally relevant MC4R mutations (out of a combined sample of 814 individuals), and found that higher rates of binge eating were not associated with these MC4R mutations. The authors report that this study had more than adequate statistical power; thus their results are not likely due to Type II error. However, Hebebrand *et al.* also note that perhaps their findings differed from those of Branson *et al.* because their assessment of binge eating was based upon a structured clinical interview, whereas the Branson *et al.* (2003) study used independent clinical interviews conducted by a dietician and a psychologist. Thus, the results of these two studies should be replicated. In addition, other candidates for binge eating should continue to be pursued.

Summary of important findings and future directions

The recent twin, family, linkage and association studies conducted in the area of EDs each make specific contributions to the field. However, some conclusions can be drawn across investigations. First, it is extremely important to study phenotypes across the lifespan, as was highlighted in the studies of Klump *et al.* (2003) and Silberg and Bulik (in press). Genes and environmental factors that influence a trait of interest may not be evident at one time point, but may be extremely important at another. Thus, both family and twin studies should scrutinize sample age with reference to age at onset and more frequently utilize longitudinal designs.

A second theme across studies is that the assessment of ED traits at the symptom level appears to provide more information about the underlying genetic and environmental structure of these disorders than diagnostic-level assessment. Several of the twin studies found distinct differences in the relative contributions of genetic and environmental factors to specific ED traits assessed at a symptom level (e.g. Neale *et al.* 2003; Reichborn-Kjennerud *et al.* 2004; Keski-Rahkonen *et al.* 2005). Only one association study (Ricca *et al.* 2004) examined ED traits at a symptom level; however, its findings indicated that symptom-level measures were uniquely associated with the polymorphism under investigation. Given that it is extremely unlikely the human genome maps directly onto DSM-IV, the refinement and elaboration of relevant phenotypes may be facilitated by studies such as these, which include measures of specific traits relevant to EDs.

In addition, the findings across twin studies also provide important information about the environment's influence on ED-related behaviors and attitudes. For example, several studies identified strong contributions of shared environment to ED-related traits (e.g. Neale *et al.* 2004; Reichborn-Kjennerud *et al.* 2004). This is noteworthy, as the ED phenotype has typically been found to be largely influenced by genetic factors. Findings identifying the relevance of the environment for specific traits are also particularly important given that the genetic epidemiology of EDs is increasingly focused on gene–environment (G × E) interactions. Thus, environmental factors identified as relevant to ED phenotypes could be further explored in G × E designs.

Clinical implications

Currently, individuals with genetic risk for certain disorders cannot change their DNA. However, this does not mean that clinicians, patients and families at risk for EDs should regard studies indicating that EDs are heritable with dismay. Rather, these data provide important information that can be used to develop prevention programs tailored for individuals most at risk for developing EDs, including the offspring of individuals with ED histories. Clinicians should emphasize that a genetic predisposition to develop an ED does not mean that expression of this predisposition is inevitable. Prevention programs could focus on teaching families at risk how to be alert for early detection and how to work towards developing buffering environments. Based on findings of the Reichborn-Kjennerud *et al.* study, self-evaluation may be a critical area for prevention programs to target, as it appears to be strongly influenced by the environment, and it can be altered. For example, parents could work actively with their children to discourage the overemphasis of weight or appearance ideals in their self-concept. In addition, parents could encourage children's participation in non-appearance focused sports and activities. Similarly, parents' modeling of healthy eating and exercise behaviors, as well as positive appearance-related attitudes, is essential, particularly in light of findings indicating that dieting is, in part, learned within the family environment (e.g. Neale *et al.* 2004). Nonetheless, even with optimal buffering family environments, individuals may still fall prey to eating disorders, and clinicians and researchers need to be vigilant to avoid placing blame (be it genetic or environmental) on parents.

Future studies should attempt to identify additional environmental targets that either directly or via various forms of gene–environment interaction or correlation influence risk for EDs. Simultaneously, additional studies identifying specific genes that influence ED susceptibility could lead to pharmacological advances that facilitate ED prevention and treatment.

Corresponding author: Cynthia M Bulik, Department of Psychiatry, University of North Carolina at Chapel Hill, CB#7160, 101 Manning Drive, Chapel Hill, NC 27599-7160, USA. Email: cbulik@med.unc.edu

References

References included from the targeted review years are preceded by one asterisk. References preceded by three asterisks are of particular significance. The significance is explained by a short commentary following the complete reference.

*Bergen AW, van den Bree MB *et al.* (2003) Candidate genes for anorexia nervosa in the 1p33-36 linkage region: serotonin 1D and delta opioid receptor loci exhibit significant association to anorexia nervosa. *Molecular Psychiatry*, **8**: 397–406.

*Branson R, Potoczna N *et al.* (2003) Binge eating as a major phenotype of melanocortin 4 receptor gene mutations. *New England Journal of Medicine*, **348**: 1096–103.

*Bulik CM, Sullivan PF and Kendle KS (2003a) Genetic and environmental contributions to obesity and binge eating. *International Journal of Eating Disorders*, **33**: 293–8.

***Bulik CM, Devlin D *et al.* (2003b) Significant linkage on chromosome 10p in families with bulimia nervosa. *American Journal of Human Genetics*, **72**: 200–7.

This paper reported significant linkage for BN on chromosome 10 (and suggestive linkage on chromosome 14), in a sample of families which include a member with BN. Interestingly, similar results were obtained when the sample was made more homogeneous by including only those families in which at least two members had purging BN (vomiting). Specifically, in the enriched subsample, the highest multipoint maximum LOD score (MLS) was on chromosome 10 between markers D10S1430 and D10S1423, and suggestive linkage was evident for chromosome 14.

Devlin B, Bacanu SA, Klump KL *et al.* (2002) Linkage analysis of anorexia nervosa incorporating behavioral covariates. *Human Molecular Genetics*, **11**: 689–96.

Di Bella DD, Catalano M, Cavaleini MC *et al.* (2000) Serotonin transporter linked polymorphic region in anorexia nervosa and bulimia nervosa. *Molecular Psychiatry*, **5**: 233–4.

*Friedel S, Horro FF, Wermter AK *et al.* (2005) Mutation screen of the brain derived neurotrophic factor gene (BDNF): identification of several genetic variants and association studies in patients with obesity, eating disorders, and attention-deficit/hyperactivity disorder. *American Journal of Medical Genetics*, **132B**: 96–9.

Frisch A, Laufer N, Danziger Y *et al.* (2001) Association of anorexia nervosa with the high activity allele of the COMT gene: a family-based study in Israeli patients. *Molecular Psychiatry*, **6**: 243–5.

*Fuentes JA, Lauzurica N, Hurtado A *et al.* (2004) Analysis of the -1438 G/A polymorphism of the 5-HT2A serotonin receptor gene in bulimia nervosa patients with or without a history of anorexia nervosa. *Psychiatric Genetics*, **14**: 107–9.

*Gabrovsek M, Brecelj-Anderluh M, Bellodi L *et al.* (2004) Combined family trio and case-control analysis of the COMT Val158Met polymorphism in European patients with anorexia nervosa. *American Journal of Medical Genetics*, **124B**: 68–72.

Grice DE, Halmi KA, Fichter MM *et al.* (2002) Evidence for a susceptibility gene for anorexia nervosa on chromosome 1. *American Journal of Human Genetics*, **70**: 787–92.

Grigoroiu-Serbanescu M, Magureanu S *et al.* (2003) Modest familial aggregation of eating disorders in restrictive anorexia nervosa with adolescent onset in a Romanian sample. *European Journal of Child and Adolescent Psychiatry*, **12**: Suppl 1:I47–53.

*Hall D, Dhilla A, Charalambous A, Gogos JA and Karayiorgou M (2003) Sequence variants of the brain-derived neurotrophic factor (BDNF) gene are strongly associated with obsessive-compulsive disorder. *American Journal of Human Genetics*, **73**: 370–6.

*Hebebrand J, Geller F, Dempfle A *et al.* (2004) Binge-eating episodes are not characteristic of carriers of melanocortin-4 receptor gene mutations. *Molecular Psychiatry*, **Aug;9(8)**: 796–800.

Heils A, Teufel A, Petri S *et al.* (1996) Allelic variation of human serotonin transporter gene expression. *Journal of Neurochemistry*, **66**: 2621–4.

Hinney A, Barth N, Ziegler A *et al.* (1997) Serotonin transporter gene-linked polymorphic region: allele distributions in relationship to body weight and in anorexia nervosa. *Life Sciences*, **61(21)**: PL295–303.

Hinney A, Remschmidt H and Hebebrand J (2000) Candidate gene polymorphisms in eating disorders. *European Journal of Pharmacology*, **410**: 147–59.

*Hu X, Giotakis O, Li T *et al.* (2003) Association of the 5-HT2c gene with susceptibility and minimum body mass index in anorexia nervosa. *Neuroreport*, **14**: 781–3.

*Hudson JI, Pope HG, Lalonde JK *et al.* (2004) Family study of binge eating disorder. Presented at the Academy for Eating Disorders Conference, Orlando, FL, April.

Kaye WH, Gwirtsman HE, George DT *et al.* (1991) Altered serotonin activity in anorexia nervosa after long-term weight recovery. *Archives of General Psychiatry*, **48**: 556–62.

Kaye WH, Nagata T, Weltzin TE *et al.* (2001) Double-blind placebo-controlled administration of fluoxetine in restricting- and restricting-purging-type anorexia nervosa. *Biological Psychiatry*, **49**: 644–52.

*Keski-Rahkonen A, Bulik CM, Neale BM *et al.* (2005) Body dissatisfaction and drive for thinness in young adult twins. *International Journal of Eating Disorders*, **37**: 188–99.

Klump KL, McGue M and Iacono WG (2000) Age differences in genetic and environmental influences on eating attitudes and behaviors in preadolescent and adolescent female twins. *Journal of Abnormal Psychology*, **109**: 239–51.

*Klump KL, McGue M and Iacono WG (2003) Differential heritability of eating attitudes and behaviors in prepubertal versus pubertal twins. *International Journal of Eating Disorders*, **33**: 287–92.

*Koizumi H, Hashimoto K, Itoh K *et al.* (2004) Association between the brain-derived neurotrophic factor 196G/A polymorphism and eating disorders. *American Journal of Medical Genetics*, **127B**: 125–7.

*Koronyo-Hamaoui M, Gak E, Stein D *et al.* (2004) CAG repeat polymorphism within the KCNN3 gene is a significant contributor to susceptibility to anorexia nervosa: a case-control study of female patients and several ethnic groups in the Israeli Jewish population. *American Journal of Medical Genetics*, **131B**: 76–80.

Kruglyak L, Daly MJ, Reeve-Daly MP *et al.* (1996) Parametric and nonparametric linkage analysis: a unified multipoint approach. *American Journal of Human Genetics* **58**: 1347–63.

*Lauzurica N, Hurtado A *et al.* (2003) Polymorphisms within the promoter and the intron 2 of the serotonin transporter gene in a population of bulimic patients. *Neuroscience Letters*, **352**: 226–30.

*Matsushita S, Suzuki K, Escarti A *et al.* (2004) Serotonin transporter regulatory region polymorphism is associated with anorexia nervosa. *American Journal of Medical Genetics*, **128B**: 114–7.

*Nakazato M, Hashimoto K, Shimizu E *et al.* (2003) Decreased levels of serum brain-derived neurotrophic factor in female patients with eating disorders. *Biological Psychiatry*, **54**: 485–90.

*Neale BM, Mazzeo SE and Bulik CM (2003) A twin study of dietary restraint, disinhibition and hunger: an examination of the eating inventory (three factor eating questionnaire). *Twin Research*, **6**: 471–8.

*Nilsson M, Naessén S, Dahlman I *et al.* (2004) Association of estrogen receptor beta gene polymorphisms with bulimic disease in women. *Molecular Psychiatry*, **9**: 28–34.

*Reichborn-Kjennerud T, Bulik CM, Kendler KS *et al.* (2003) Gender differences in binge-eating: a population-based twin study. *Acta Psychiatrica Scandinavica*, **108**: 196–202.

***Reichborn-Kjennerud T, Bulik CM, Kendler KS *et al.* (2004) Undue influence of weight on self-evaluation: a population-based twin study of gender differences. *International Journal of Eating Disorders*, **35**: 123–32.

This paper found that the undue influence of weight in self-evaluation was influenced by both genetic and environmental factors in both men and women. This finding regarding the importance of environmental factors is relatively rare in the area of EDs, which has previously found that many ED behaviors, such as vomiting, are highly heritable. However, the current findings provide some important directions for prevention research.

*Ribasés M, Gratacòs M, Armengol L *et al.* (2003) Met66 in the brain-derived neurotrophic factor (BDNF) precursor is associated with anorexia nervosa restrictive type. *Molecular Psychiatry*, **8**: 745–51.

*Ribasés M, Gratacòs M, Fernandez-Aranda F *et al.* (2004) Association of BDNF with anorexia, bulimia, and age of onset of weight loss in six European populations. *Human Molecular Genetics,* **13**: 1205–12.

***Ribasés M, Gratacòs M, Fernandez-Aranda F *et al.* (2005) Association of BDNF with restricting anorexia nervosa and minimum body mass index: a family-based association study of eight European populations. *European Journal of Human Genetics,* **13**: 428–34.

This investigation used a TDT approach and a multi-site recruitment strategy to examine the relevance of BDNF to EDs. Thus, its findings provide perhaps the strongest evidence to date of the association between the Met66 variant and AN-R.

*Ricca V, Nacmias B, Boldrini M *et al.* (2004) Psychopathological traits and 5-HT(2A) receptor promoter polymorphism (-1438 G/A) in patients suffering from anorexia nervosa and bulimia nervosa. *Neuroscience Letters,* **365**: 92–6.

Schulze TG and McMahon FJ (2002) Genetic association mapping at the crossroads: which test and why? Overview and practical guidelines. *American Journal of Medical Genetics,* **114**: 1–11.

*Shinohara M, Mizushima H, Hirans M *et al.* (2004) Eating disorders with binge-eating behavior are associated with the s allele of the 3′-UTR VNTR polymorphism of the dopamine transporter gene. *Journal of Psychiatry and Neuroscience,* **29**: 134–7.

*Siegfried Z, Kanyas K, Latzer Y *et al.* (2004) Association study of cannabinoid receptor gene (CNR1) alleles and anorexia nervosa: differences between restricting and binging/purging subtypes. *American Journal of Medical Genetics,* **125B**: 126–30.

***Silberg JL and Bulik CM (in press) The developmental association between eating disorders symptoms and symptoms of depression and anxiety in juvenile twin girls. *Journal of Child Psychology and Psychiatry.*

These investigators examined genetic and environmental factors associated with depression, anxiety and EDs in two cohorts of twin girls: ages 8–13 and 14–17. They found distinct differences between the two groups with respect to the factors contributing to each disorder at the two time periods measured. These findings emphasize the importance of repeated measurement of genetic and environmental susceptibilities. Moreover, they further support the link between EDs and anxiety disorders.

Slagboom PE and Meulenbelt I (2002) Organisation of the human genome and our tools for identifying disease genes. *Biological Psychology,* **61**: 11–31.

*Steiger H, Joober R, Israël M, Young SN *et al.* (2005) The 5HTTLPR polymorphism, psychopathological symptoms, and platelet [^{3}H-] paroxetine binding in bulimic syndromes. *International Journal of Eating Disorders,* **37**: 57–60.

Sullivan PF, Bulik CM and Kendler KS (1998) The genetic epidemiology of binging and vomiting. *British Journal of Psychiatry,* **173**: 75–9.

Sundaramurthy D, Pieri LF, Gape H *et al.* (2000) Analysis of the serotonin transporter gene linked polymorphism (5-HTTLPR) in anorexia nervosa. *American Journal of Medical Genetics,* **96**: 53–5.

***Urwin RE, Bennetts BH, Wilcken B *et al.* (2003a) Investigation of epistasis between the serotonin transporter and norepinephrine transporter genes in anorexia nervosa. *Neuropsychopharmacology,* **28**: 1351–5.

This study evaluated the hypothesis that the SERT and NET genes interact (i.e. are in epistasis) to cause AN. Although their results did not provide evidence of epistasis, the authors' innovative design suggests important future directions for genetic researchers, as it is likely that complex behaviors are influenced by epistatic effects.

*Urwin RE, Bennetts BH, Wilcken B *et al.* (2003b) Gene-gene interaction between the monoamine oxidase A gene and solute carrier family 6 (neurotransmitter transporter, noradrenalin) member 2 gene in anorexia nervosa (restrictive subtype). *European Journal of Human Genetics*, **11**: 945–50.

Wade T, Martin NG and Tiggemann M (1998) Genetic and environmental risk factors for the weight and shape concerns characteristic of bulimia nervosa. *Psychological Medicine*, **28**: 761–71.

3

Sociocultural issues and eating disorders

Anne E Becker and Kristen Fay

Abstract

Objectives of review. This review encompasses new epidemiologic and ethnographic data linking ethnicity, culture and socioeconomic factors to risk for eating disorders in selected papers published between 2003 and early 2005. Experimental and observational studies investigating the relation of specific social environmental influences such as mass media and family and peer environment on risk are also reviewed.

Summary of recent findings. Several recent studies suggest that prevalence across ethnic groups in the US may be similar, although several studies find disparities in prevalence. Epidemiologic studies suggest that eating disorders may have increasingly global distribution. Empirically supported models for pathogenesis of eating disorders continue to emphasize the causal role of social pressures to be thin as well as influence of mass media, and peer and family environment.

Future directions. A number of substantial methodologic limitations continue to pose challenges to interpretation of how sociocultural processes moderate etiologic pathways for eating disorders. Broader use of qualitative approaches is advocated to refine and reframe some of the research questions linking sociocultural processes to risk.

Introduction

The range of potential sociocultural influences on body image and eating disorders is broad and includes local cultural patterning of diversity in body ideals, motivation and behavior. As such, local and global cultural influences impact on both incidence and clinical phenomenology of the eating disorders. The earliest research on this topic–largely observational population studies– suggested cross-national and cross-ethnic differences in the prevalence and clinical presentation of disordered eating. More recent research has included experimental studies that have begun to elucidate etiologic pathways. An early model relating social context to disordered eating emphasized cultural valuation of thinness and its potential promotion of body dissatisfaction and disordered eating (Garner *et al.* 1980; Striegel-Moore *et al.* 1986; Stice and Shaw 1994). More recent refinements of this model include the Dual-Pathway Model of Bulimic Pathology (Stice 2001) and the Tripartite Influence Model of body image and eating disturbance (Van den Berg *et al.* 2002). In addition, there are emerging data over the past two decades that support the association of disordered eating with cultural transitioning and globalizing political and economic forces (Nasser 1986; Bendall *et al.* 1991; Mumford *et al.* 1991; Lee 1996; Davis and Katzman 1999; Nasser *et al.* 2001; Becker 2003). Both lines of inquiry have promoted understanding of how social environment contributes to risk for eating disorders. Identification of modifiable risk factors will be critical to the development of culturally sensitive and effective preventive and therapeutic interventions.

In this chapter, we review recent publications that report new epidemiologic data on the comparative prevalence of eating disorders across ethnically and culturally diverse populations and that investigate the impact of local and global cultures on risk. We also review studies investigating the relation of specific social environmental influences such as mass media and family and peer environment on risk. Studies were selected for relevance to this topic after identification through searches of the computerized databases *Medline*, *PsychINFO* and *ERIC*. Papers with primary search terms relating to eating disorders in the title (e.g. eating, body ideal, weight concern, body dissatisfaction, anorexia, bulimia, etc.) and secondary search terms relating to sociocultural factors in the title or abstract (e.g. acculturation, interpersonal, ethnic, peer, media, etc.), published in the English language between 2002 and early 2005 and involving human subjects or human populations, were examined. This review is restricted to studies published after 2002, unless a study prior to 2003 made significant and unique contributions to understanding sociocultural issues and eating disorders through important data or a novel approach, or is historically relevant to this review. Using these criteria and after reviewing content, over 110 publications were considered for inclusion.

Ethnicity and contributions to risk

Several epidemiologic studies prior to the timeframe of this review have suggested disparities in incidence of eating disorders among different ethnic groups in the United States (Anderson-Fye and Becker 2003). Notable findings from previous studies included that the presentation of symptoms associated with eating disorders was somewhat heterogeneous across ethnic groups and that certain symptom patterns appeared to be as common or more common among underserved minority women in the United States compared with White, non-Latina women. These data were critical in countering longstanding stereotypes about this illness being associated with affluence and 'White ethnicity'. In contrast, several large-scale studies in the past two years have reported data suggesting that prevalences of eating disorders across different ethnic groups may be quite similar. For example, in one large cross-sectional study (n=785), Shaw et al. (2004) found no differences among ethnic minority groups studied (Asians, Blacks, Hispanics and Whites) with respect to mean levels of any eating disorder symptoms. Similarly, Cachelin et al. (2003) found that dieting and restraint scores did not significantly differ among Asian, Latino and White adolescent girls and boys (n=211). Finally, a study of obese bariatric surgery candidates (n=210) reported an absence of significant differences in prevalences of binge eating or BED in White versus ethnic minority (African American and Latina) women (Sanchez-Johnson et al. 2003).

Shaw and colleagues (2004) suggest that prevalence rates may be converging due to the homogenization of cultural influences on body image and eating disturbances. However, it is not clear whether actual incidence is changing or whether previous estimates have been biased. Moreover, some data do suggest continued disparities. Most notably, a large prospective cohort study (n=2046) found that Black women were less likely than White women to have an eating disorder. Moreover, marginally significantly fewer Black women met criteria for BED than White women (i.e. 1.4% of Black women vs. 2.7% of White women; OR=2.0, 95% CI 1.0–3.8)–a finding contradictory to previous studies (Striegel-Moore et al. 2003). This study and the Sanchez-Johnson study are consistent in disconfirming that Black women have a higher prevalence of BED than White women in the United States. In addition, a cross-sectional comparison of school-age girls with the EAT-26 and CHEAT demonstrated that Native American respondents scored significantly higher on the restricting/purging and dieting factors than either Whites or non-White/non-Native Americans, after adjusting for age and BMI (Lynch et al. 2004). Finally, a meta-analysis of 18 published studies (over the period 1987–2001) evaluating the comparative prevalence of eating disturbances among African American and White women also found that African American women have fewer eating disturbances than do White women (O'Neill 2003).

In addition to prevalence studies, a number of reports strongly suggest cross-ethnic variation in values and perceptions relating to self and body image, believed to be pertinent to disordered eating. For example, in a study of college women, Blacks perceived a significantly different and larger body ideal for themselves than did Whites (Perez and Joiner 2003). Similarly, African American men preferred significantly larger body size for women than their White counterparts (Freedman et al. 2004). Likewise, a comparison of African American and Caucasian adolescent girls revealed that African American girls held more favorable attitudes about physical appearance, reported less social pressures for thinness, and less tendency to base self-esteem on body-related factors than did Caucasian girls (White *et al.* 2003).

By contrast, a study of elementary schoolgirls found that non-Caucasian (i.e. Black, Latino, Asian and mixed ethnicity) girls reported significantly greater internalization of a thin ideal than non-Hispanic, White girls (Hermes and Keel 2003). These seemingly contradictory results raise the question of whether perceived social and economic disadvantage may sensitize girls and women towards culturally dominant body ideals and ultimately impact on pathogenesis of disordered eating. For instance, a study of 122 American college-age women of south Asian descent found that racial teasing, but not ethnic identification or acculturation measures, was significantly associated with body dissatisfaction and disturbed eating (Iyer and Haslam 2003). Finally, another potentially fruitful avenue of research has taken a broader perspective on which dimensions of self-presentation are most culturally salient. A qualitative study of college-educated African American and Latina women suggested that an ethic of grooming and self-care was emphasized over a specific body type in self-presentation (Rubin *et al.* 2003).

Ethnic-specific variation in risk for disordered eating raises new questions about resilience and vulnerability. On the one hand, there are data to suggest that differences in body ideals, interest in body esthetics (versus body care), and in self-perception in relation to these ideals, may result in less body dissatisfaction and perhaps lower risk of disordered eating. By contrast, data suggesting an association between acculturation and social transition across diverse social contexts (Becker 2003) suggest that interfacing with new images and values may increase risk. These protective and risk factors may exert divergent or overlapping effects depending on other geographic, social, or economic factors. Therefore, a convergence in prevalence of disordered eating also does not imply an absence of ethnicity-specific etiologic pathways to eating disorders.

In addition to differences in measured prevalence of disordered eating, ethnic disparities in access to care for eating disorders are of special concern. One study has found that Afro-American women are significantly less likely to receive care for an eating disorder (Cachelin *et al.* 2001) and another has found that Latina and Native American college students are significantly less likely to receive a referral for care compared with non-Latinos, when adjusting for severity of illness (Becker *et al.* 2003). Although differences in help-seeking patterns cannot be excluded, the former study suggested that symptomatic ethnic minority women were less likely to be queried by a doctor about symptoms than non-minority women. Moreover, an experimental study demonstrated that a fictional patient with Hispanic or Afro-American ethnicity was less likely to have eating disorder symptoms recognized by subjects (Gordon *et al.* 2002). Such findings suggest the importance of educating clinicians about potential clinical biases that might undermine detection of eating disorders in ethnic minority patients.

Transcultural studies in non-Western societies

Several new studies reporting data on the prevalence of disordered eating and related attitudes in Africa, Asia, the Pacific, eastern Europe, the Caribbean, and Central and South America represent important progress in identifying the global distribution of eating disorders (*see* Table 3.1). Of special interest in transcultural comparisons are phenomenologic disparities in disordered eating. For example, British south Asian adolescents are less likely to present with fat phobia compared with British White adolescents (Tareen *et al.* 2005). Similarly, drive for thinness is significantly lower among Japanese treatment-seeking women with eating disorders in Tokyo as compared with North American women (Pike and Mizushima 2005). Finally, a study found that Taiwanese men have significantly less body dissatisfaction than American men (Yang *et al.* 2005). By contrast, a case series of five men with eating disorders in central China described fear of fatness in all cases (Tong *et al.* 2005). The variation in findings suggests that cultural influences on body image may be quite dynamic.

Acculturation and risk for eating disorders

From the 1980s through the past few years, a number of epidemiologic studies have suggested that social transition may increase risk for disordered eating among vulnerable individuals. For example, in studies of young women from south Asia, Egypt, Pakistan and Greece, risk for disordered eating has been observed to be higher in populations experiencing transnational migration than in those in their country of origin (Becker 2003). Moreover, both modernization and exposure to Western products, images, ideas and values appear to contribute to risk as well–albeit via mechanisms that are incompletely understood. An extensive review by Keel and Klump (2003) concluded that no reported cases of BN in the transcultural literature occurred in the absence of exposure to Western culture (notably, they did not find this to be true for AN). This impact–often glossed as acculturation–has been the subject of many additional studies, although the term is often loosely or inconsistently defined. Moreover, its operationalization as a predictor of risk has been challenging because the dimensions and impact of acculturation are relative to their specific cultural context.

Recent studies suggesting a positive association between acculturation and disordered eating include one by Bhugra and Bhui (2003) that found that Black middle school students in East London who wore English clothing were significantly more likely to have highest quartile Bulimic Investigatory Test-Edinburgh (BITE) scores. Similarly, there was a marginally significant association between non-White, non-Black and non-Asian students who read in English only and also scored in the highest quartile (Bhugra and Bhui 2003). Likewise, Asian adolescent girls who scored higher on the Suinn-Lew Asian Self-Identity-Acculturation Scale (AL-ASIA) were significantly more likely to be dieters than those with lower scores (Cachelin *et al.* 2003).

Other findings support that the effects of ethnic identification, assimilation and acculturation on disordered eating may be highly situation specific, as well

Table 3.1   Selected transcultural studies assessing disturbance in body image and eating

Study	Geographical regions	Study population	Recruitment	ED specific instruments	Instrument validated? Translated?	Main ED outcome measured	Selected findings
Baranowski et al. (2003)	Scotland and Yugoslavia	n=625 Adolescent boys and girls from: Dundee, Scotland (n=325; M=13 yrs) and Belgrade, Yugoslavia (n=303; M=12 yrs)	School-based (urban)	-Contour Drawing Rating Scale -Body-Cathexis Scale (7 items) -BSQ -DEBQ-Restraint item -TFEQ-Disinhibition item -CHEAT	Not reported	-Body dissatisfaction -Restrained eating -Disinhibition (overeating) -Dieting history	-Eating pathology and body dissatisfaction higher among Scottish cohort, and particularly in Scottish girls (all p<.05)
Becker et al. (2003)	Fiji	n=50 Adult ethnic Fijian females in rural Fiji	Community	QEWP-R	Translated into Nadroga language/ backtranslated with consultation of local informants	Binge eating Binge-eating disorder	4% met DSM criteria for BED 10% had binge episodes at least weekly

Table 3.1   Continued

Bennett *et al.* (2004)	Ghana	*n*=668 Female students in rural Ghana (median=18 yrs)	School-based (rural)	-EAT-40 -BITE	-EAT validated in W African population (Oyewumi and Kazarin 1992) -Study conducted in English as semi-structured interview	-Anorexic-like behavior (total score cutoff EAT≥30) -Bulimic symptoms (total score cutoff BITE≥25)	-Only 10 (1.5%) with BMI<17.5 appeared to have self-starvation as cause of low weight -All 10 viewed restriction positively and religiously w/o typical AN weight-related concerns
Bhugra *et al.* (2003)	Trinidad and Barbados	*n*=362 girls (M=15 yrs) 26% Indian 53% African 19% (White, mixed)	School-based	-BITE -DSM-IIR Bulimic Diagnostic Interview (25% of total sample randomly selected) -Questionnaire developed for this study	English version of questionnaire used	-Clinical and sub-clinical cases -Bulimic symptoms (symptom and severity cutoff scores) -Concern with weight and shape (DSM-IIR BDI)	-Only .8% of subjects scored above BITE cut-off and no interviewees could be diagnosed with BN -African girls, relative to Indian and 'Other,' more often believed food dominated their life (*p*=.007) and worried they had no control over amount they ate (*p*=.009)

Table 3.1   Continued

Study	Geographical regions	Study population	Recruitment	ED specific instruments	Instrument validated? Translated?	Main ED outcome measured	Selected findings
Bilukha and Utermohlen (2002)	Ukraine	*n*=616 Women from Lviv City (M=28 yrs)	School- and community-based (urban)	-SATAQ -Stunkard's Nine-Figure scale -Dieting history-prior 6 months	-Not reported -Translated into Ukrainian and then back-translated	-Desire to achieve Western ideal of thinness -Figure dissatisfaction	-Western media exposure related to internalization (*p*<.0001) -Increased dieting risk among younger women, overweight women, and those who desired Western ideal figure (*p*<.0001 for all)
Bojorquez and Unikel (2004)	Mexico	*n*=458 Teenage girls in Michoacan, Mexico (M=16.5 yrs)	School-based (semi-urban and small urban)	-EDI -Risk eating behaviors checklist	-EDI-Spanish version (Garner 1998), validated in Mexico (Alvarez and Paredes 2001)	-ED-risk level -Algorithim based on endorsed behaviors/ attitudes	1.7% potential at risk for eating disorder

Table 3.1   Continued

Edman and Yates (2004)	Guam California	59 Chamorro (M=26 yrs) 76 Caucasian (M=25 yrs) female students	School-based (urban)	-EDI-2 (DT, IA, IE subscales) -Stunkard's Nine-Figure scale -Self-Loathing subscale (SLSS)	-Not reported -All instruments administered in English, official language	-ED-risk level -Body dissatisfaction	No significant ethnic differences on EDI-2, body dissatisfaction, and SLSS scores
Hawks et al. (2003)	Japan Western US	n=1218 College men and women in Japan (M=21 yrs) and United States (M=yrs)	School-based (one college in Japan, two in US)	-Motivation for Eating Scale (MFES) -General questions related to dieting, exercise, and disordered eating history	-Not reported -Translated into Japanese, and pilot tested for understanding	-Motivation for eating (emotional, physical, environmental)	-No significant differences in three MFES subscales for men in US and Japan -US women more likely to eat for emotional (p=.002) reasons, while women in Japan more likely to eat for physical (p=.008) or environmental (p<.0001) reasons
Nunes et al. (2003)	Brazil	n=513 Women in Porto Alegre, Brazil (M=20 yrs)	Community-based	-EAT-26 -BITE	-Not reported -Trained interviewers	Used various cutoff points to operationalize	-10.9% with abnormal eating behaviors 23.8% unusual

Table 3.1 Continued

Study	Geographical regions	Study population	Recruitment	ED specific instruments	Instrument validated? Translated?	Main ED outcome measured	Selected findings
					administered EAT/BITE given low educational levels	BITE/EAT scores into three groups: 1) abnormal eating; 2) unusual eating; 3) normal eating	eating patterns; 60.2% normal eating behaviors -Abnormal eating behaviors more prevalent among higher-BMI women ($p=.009$)
Tölgyes and Nemessury (2004)	Budapest and Pécs	$n=580$ Secondary school and college females and males in Budapest ($n=340$) and Pécs (240). Age range 10–29 yrs	School-based	-BITE -EAT-40 -SCID-DSM-IV	-BITE translated into Hungarian -BITE only validated in English-speaking countries but carried out pilot study based on translation -EAT translated and standardized (Túry et al. 1990)	-At-risk -EAT>29 (cutoff anorexic disposition) -BITE>25 (cutoff total score)	-3% revealed AN disposition, but no actual cases (BMI<17.5) -4.5% of females and .8% males classified as subclinical BN, and 3.6% of females and .4% of males listed as simulated BN -.6% prevalence of BN proved by diagnostic interview

as multifaceted. For example, ethnic identity was also found to moderate the effect of parental and peer influences on body image in Chinese women residing in Australia, such that stronger ethnic identification was associated with greater eating pathology when the respondent also reported overprotection by the parent. By contrast, weaker ethnic identification was associated with greater eating pathology in the setting of greater feedback from father or male friend about weight or body shape (Humphrey and Ricciardelli 2004). Another study illustrates an inverse association between acculturation and disordered eating. A large comparative study of Taiwanese women (*n*=347) and Taiwanese-American women (*n*=305) found that Taiwanese-American respondents were less traditional than Taiwanese respondents and also had significantly less body dissatisfaction and disordered eating attitudes and behaviors. Moreover, among the Taiwanese-American group, lower ethnic identification was significantly associated with lower body dissatisfaction and disordered eating (Tsai *et al.* 2003).

Several qualitative studies exploring the relation of cultural change to body image and disordered eating have indeed suggested that the response to social transition varies. For example, among Belizean adolescent girls, rapid economic and social change does not appear to be associated with an increased prevalence of eating disorders (Anderson-Fye 2004). Of particular interest are ethnographic data that suggest that indigenous ideals concerning bodily dimensions other than size or weight may have a protective role. For example, in Belize, girls and women are more interested in shape (i.e. curvaceousness is valued) than in size (Anderson-Fye 2004). Moreover, in Papua-New Guinea, girls with greater television exposure did not wish to pursue a thinner body ideal, although they indicated a wish to be taller compared with girls with less exposure (Wesch 2004).

In other settings, qualitative data support an association between social change and disturbances in body image and eating. For example, a meticulous study of incident cases of AN in Curacao found cases only among mixed ethnicity women. Of interest here, these women consistently reported their perception that thinness allowed them greater acceptance in the more affluent, White community (Katzman *et al.* 2004). Similarly, ethnic Fijian secondary-school girls in Fiji reported an explicit desire to emulate television characters' body shape and size partly in relation to a pragmatic desire to expand economic opportunities. Notwithstanding the underlying motivation to lose weight, these efforts did occasionally result in eating pathology (Becker 2004). In these latter two examples, disordered eating was associated with the perception that reshaping the body would allow upward social mobility. Ethnographic data from Japan suggest that eating pathology there may be linked to perceived conflict between traditional and modernizing roles for women (Pike and Borovoy 2004). In each of these studies, the pursuit of thinness is observed to be secondary or incidental to other motivations. These ethnographic data suggest the sociocultural contributions to risk and resilience may differ substantially within the local cultural contexts. For this reason, a simple model for sociocultural mediation of pathogenesis is unlikely.

Contributions of the social environment to risk

Empirically supported models relating social environment to disordered eating have emphasized social pressures to be thin, internalization of a thin ideal, and body dissatisfaction as precursors to disordered eating (e.g. Stice 2002; Van den Berg *et al.* 2002). Therefore, there are multiple points at which both local and global sociocultural environments may buffer or exacerbate elements of the etiologic pathways to an eating disorder.

Social comparison and mediation of disordered eating

A chief investigative focus has been how social comparison (Festinger 1954) may promote body dissatisfaction and disordered eating. This has motivated multiple studies on media, peer and family influence on risk for eating disorders. On the other hand, consistent effects of social comparison on disordered eating across culturally distinct populations are unlikely. Not only is there cross-cultural diversity in body ideals, but in how the response to these ideals is patterned. For example, social comparison will be likely to motivate behavior and impact on self-evaluation and body image differently depending on dimensions of self-presentation and/or appearance deemed most socially valuable, perceived personal responsibility for the body, autonomy, and endorsement of competition and achievement.

Several studies in the past two years have expanded our understanding of how social comparison may promote risk for disordered eating but have yielded more questions than answers. Data from these studies suggest that the effects of social comparison may be mediated by mood and additional information, that social comparison of appearance may be relevant within specific strata of socioeconomic status (SES), and that additional dimensions of social comparison (i.e. in addition to appearance-related comparison) may impact upon disordered eating. One recent study did demonstrate that patients with eating disorders, as compared to a healthy control group, make significantly less favorable comparisons with others (Troop *et al.* 2003). By contrast, another cross-sectional study did not find that female outpatients with confirmed diagnoses of eating disorders were significantly different from a non-clinical sample of female college students on assessments of social comparison (Morrison *et al.* 2003). This finding is noteworthy since it is counter to expectations under the hypothesis that social comparison leads to body dissatisfaction that may contribute to risk for eating disorders. More data are required before conclusions can be drawn.

A cross-sectional study of female university students suggested that depression may also moderate the effect of social comparison and social anxiety on disordered eating (Gilbert and Meyer 2003). In addition, Evans (2003) reported data from an experimental study suggesting that the association of thinness with positive life success may play an important role in mediating the effects of social comparison. In this study, respondents (US female university students) who received stereotype-disconfirming information about the thin stimulus image reported significantly higher optimism about future life, mood, and higher appearance and social state self-esteem when compared with those who received stereotype-confirming information. These results suggest that assisting young women in deconstructing media images may have a role in prevention strategies for eating disorders. Further examination of the multiple dimensions of social comparison will be instrumental to understanding how socially mediated body ideals, social comparison and hierarchy may relate to disordered eating. For example, Troop and colleagues (2003) identified three factors in the Social Comparison Rating Scale (SCRS) that included social comparison of rank, of group fit and of appearance. The former two may be especially relevant effect modifiers among populations of women who may perceive themselves as socially marginalized, such as immigrant or socially disadvantaged populations.

The influence of mass media exposure on body image and disordered eating

Continued evidence (Voracek and Fisher 2002; Sypeck *et al.* 2004) supports increasingly thin beauty ideals during the past 40 years. The transmission of these cultural ideals by Western media images and messages has been associated with body dissatisfaction, disordered eating, weight concerns and unhealthy weight control methods (Hargreaves and Tiggemann 2003a; Frisby 2004). Numerous observational and experimental studies have continued to support the association between media exposure and disordered eating. Our review of the literature identified nine experimental studies–including six randomized controlled trials–and eight observational studies on the impact of media on body image and disordered eating (*see* Table 3.2). Overall the majority of these studies were in agreement in finding an adverse effect of the media on body image, eating attitudes and behaviors.

Among the randomized controlled trials supporting an adverse effect of media exposure on body image, Tiggemann and Slater (2004) found brief exposure to music videos containing thin and attractive images of women led to increased social comparison and body dissatisfaction. In another experiment, Halliwell and Dittmar (2004) randomly assigned female subjects to view print advertisements of thin models, average models, or no models. Among women who internalize thin appearance ideals, viewing pictures of thin models induced greater weight-related appearance concerns than exposure to average-size models or no models (Halliwell and Dittmar 2004). Murnen *et al.* (2003) found an increased awareness of and desire to emulate unrealistic bodily standards among grade-school girls and boys exposed to pictures of objectified men and women. In one study among college women, watching TV with relatively more White cast members was linked to increased bulimic tendencies among Black women. Among White respondents, this was associated with greater body dissatisfaction (Schooler *et al.* 2004). While the majority of studies (Groesz *et al.* 2002; Hausenblas *et al.* 2004) have evaluated the short-term effects of media exposure on body image and disordered eating, one innovative experiment (Hargreaves and Tiggemann 2003b) found that adolescent girls exposed to

Table 3.2 Experimental studies assessing the relation of media exposure to body dissatisfaction and disordered eating

Study	Study aim	Study population	Study design	Assessments	Key findings
Halliwell and Dittmar (2004)	Examine effect of types of print ads featuring thin, average-size, or no models on women's body image	Caucasian, non-student women in the UK (n=202)	RCT **Exposure:** Print ads of thin models, average models, or no models	-Sociocultural attitudes toward appearance questionnaire (SATAQ) -Physical appearance state and trait anxiety scale (PASTAS)	-Exposure to thin models related to increased body-focused anxiety among women who internalize the thin ideal than exposure to average-size models or no models (p<.01)
Hargreaves and Tiggemann (2003a)	Investigate effect of viewing televised images of female attractiveness on adolescents' body dissatisfaction	160 girls and 197 boys from Australian high school (n=357)	RCT **Exposure:** 20 appearance- or 20 non-appearance-related commercials	-Visual analogue scales (VAS)- body dissatisfaction -Word-stem completion task -Appearance schemas inventory	-Girls, but not boys, who viewed appearance commercials reported higher body dissatisfaction relative to non-appearance condition (p<.001) -Both boys and girls in appearance condition reported greater appearance-related thoughts (p<.001)

Table 3.2   Continued

Hargreaves and Tiggemann (2003b)	Examine relationship between immediate responses to media images and the development of body dissatisfaction over 2-year time period	42 girls and 38 boys from Australian high school (*n*=80) in Year 10 (Time 1) and Year 12 (Time 2)	RCT **Exposure:** 20 appearance- or 20 non-appearance-related commercials	-VAS-body dissatisfaction -EDI-drive for thinness -Drive for muscularity (based on EDI-DT)	-For girls, appearance commercials significantly related to increased T1 and T2 body dissatisfaction (*p*<.001) and drive for thinness (*p*<.01) scores -Similar results observed for boys' drive for thinness but not body dissatisfaction (*p*<.05)
Hausenblas *et al.* (2004)	Examine the affective responses of media exposure for women either high or low on drive for thinness (DT)	Caucasian female university students (*n*=30)	RCT **Exposure:** 8 full-body self slides; 8 full-body model slides, and 8 non-body control slides	-EDI-2 (body dissatisfaction, bulimia, and drive for thinness) -Positive and negative affect scale (PANAS)	-Higher-DT group, compared to the lower-DT group, reported less pleasure while viewing the self slides, more negative affect immediately after viewing the self slides and one and two hours after viewing the model slides (*p*<.05 for all)

Table 3.2   Continued

Study	Study aim	Study population	Study design	Assessments	Key findings
Murnen *et al.* (2003)	Examine young children's responses to objectified images of women and men	Caucasian, grade school girls (*n*=88) and boys (*n*=58) in rural Ohio	Cross-sectional experiment **Exposure:** 4 male and 4 female model images	-SATAQ -BES -Asked for responses to photos	-Among girls, greater thin ideal awareness related to increased desire to emulate model (*p*<.001) -For boys, internalization, but not awareness, related to wanting to look like models (*p*<.001)
Tiggemann and Slater (2004)	Investigate the impact of idealized female images in music television	Female college students at Flinders University in Australia (*n*=84)	RCT **Exposure:** Appearance- or non-appearance-related music videos	-VAS-Mood and body dissatisfaction -Appearance and comparison processing questions	-Viewing appearance music videos led to increased social comparison and body dissatisfaction (*p*<.05)
Becker *et al.* (2002)	Assess impact of novel, prolonged television exposure on disordered eating attitudes and behaviors among ethnic Fijian adolescent girls	Adolescent ethnic Fijian girls from two secondary schools in Nadroga, Fiji (*n*=63 at T1 and *n*=65 at T2)	Naturalistic experiment **Exposure:** Western Media Imagery-TV (1998 cohort)	-Modified EAT-26 -Questions about TV viewing and household ownership -Semi-structured interview to confirm weight control behaviors	-Key indicators of disordered eating more prevalent following exposure -Narrative data reflected interest in weight loss to emulate TV characters

Table 3.2 Continued

Frisby (2004)	Examine impact of exposure to advertisements of thin, attractive Caucasian and Afro-American models on self-evaluations of Afro-American women	African American college females (*n*=110)	Cross-sectional experiment **Exposure:** 10 experimental (Afro-American or Caucasian model) and 10 filler (product) ads	-Body Esteem Scale (BES) -Transient mood state	-Exposure to Caucasian images did not significantly impact self-esteem (*p*>.7) -Exposure to African-American models negatively affects Black women who are less satisfied with their bodies (*p*<.05)
Joshi *et al.* (2004)	Examine the effect of thin-body media images on mood, self-esteem, and self-image ratings of restrained and unrestrained eaters	University of Toronto female undergraduate students (*n*=92)	RCT **Exposure:** Thin-body model ads and control product ads	-Current thoughts scale -Self-image scale -Affect rating scale (ARS) -Restraint scale	-Exposure to thin images among restrained eaters was related to improved self-image (*p*<.07) and social self-esteem (*p*<.03) -Unrestrained eaters showed decreased appearance self-esteem after viewing too thin images (*p*<.004)

commercials depicting thin, attractive models reported feeling more dissatisfied with their bodies and expressed greater drive for thinness two years later.

Overall, observational and experimental data provide cumulative support for a causal effect of mass media exposure in the development of longer term body image disturbance. They also suggest several pathways through which media images threaten self- and body-esteem. In his dual-pathway model, Stice (2001 and 2002) demonstrated that internalization of these unrealistic media ideals heightens levels of body dissatisfaction and increases risk for bulimic pathology. Several recent studies have further supported the media's adverse impact on vulnerable individuals through internalization of these cultural norms (Van den Berg *et al.* 2002; Blowers *et al.* 2003). For example, Low and colleagues (2003) found that internalization of the thin ideal, not awareness of it, was immediately and prospectively associated with increased eating and weight concerns among college women. Thus internalization of the cultural valuation of leanness and attractiveness negatively impacts body dissatisfaction and increases risk of disordered eating; similar effects are observed across a variety of age, gender and ethnic groups.

Observational and experimental studies on media effects have some vexing limitations–the former because of challenges in drawing causal inference and the latter due to a lack of both ecological validity and of unexposed populations. By contrast, a natural experiment investigating the impact of the introduction of Western media imagery to rural Fiji–where the prevalence of eating disorders was extremely low and the valuation of robust body shape comparatively high– suggested a causal association between television exposure and increased disordered eating attitudes and behaviors among adolescent girls (Becker *et al.* 2002). In a related study, narrative data strongly suggested that Fijian girls perceived their social and economic opportunities would be enhanced by weight loss (Becker 2004). In this cultural context, the media not only promoted the social value of slimness but also encouraged dietary restraint and body reshaping as a strategy for social and economic advancement.

Not all studies have found conclusive support for the direct impact of media images on the development of problematic eating, suggesting that the relation is not always straightforward (Fouts and Vaughan 2002; Joshi *et al.* 2004). For example, in a study of adolescent girls, Fouts and Vaughan (2002) found no main effect of television exposure on disordered eating but, instead, found a moderating effect for (internal vs. external) locus of control such that those girls who viewed more television and showed an internal locus of control reported less disordered eating compared to those with an external locus of control. Similarly, in an investigation of college females, exposure to thin media images led to increased positive self-image and social self-esteem among restrained eaters and decreased appearance self-esteem among unrestrained eaters (Joshi *et al.* 2004). In addition, some data suggest that mass media may have varying effects on consumers. For example, among female undergraduate students, the relationship between magazine exposure–but not television exposure–and body dissatisfaction was mediated by internalization of thin ideals (Tiggemann 2003).

Peer influence

Outside the cultural sphere of influence, several lines of evidence suggest that localized social networks and 'subcultures', such as schools, neighborhoods and peer groups, transmit and reinforce social norms and values that perpetuate risk for body dissatisfaction and eating pathology (Lin and Kulik 2002; Presnell *et al.* 2004). For example, higher rates of eating disorders and weight concerns are reported among populations involved in sport activities in which leanness is valued and encouraged, such as dance, swimming, gymnastics, cheerleading (Davison *et al.* 2002; Thompson and Digsby 2004). In a recent study of sorority and non-sorority women, sorority women maintained more rigorous dietary attitudes and behaviors over the course of their college education (Allison and Park 2004). Wardle and Watters (2004) found that among 9- and 11-year-old girls, greater exposure to older peers in school was associated with increased weight concern, dieting and thinner size ideals. The preceding data suggest that exposure to peer networks that emphasize slimness and dietary restraint contributes to the risk for the development of eating disorders.

Weight- and appearance-specific social norms within adolescents' proximal peer networks have been identified as strong predictors of weight concerns and restrained eating (Van den Berg *et al.* 2002; Neumark-Sztainer *et al.* 2003). In a nationwide survey of adolescent health, Kaltiala-Heino and colleagues (2003) found less frequent perceptions of being overweight among respondents. They used these findings to refute public debate surrounding cultural valuation of thinness and suggest, instead, that adolescents more often engage in evaluation against their peers than against societal esthetic ideals. Moreover, a large cross-sectional study of secondary schoolgirls in northern England found that girls from higher SES social environments reported significantly greater exposure to weight loss and dieting (e.g. family and friends engaged in weight loss behaviors and discussion). Higher SES girls in this study also indicated a greater awareness of ideals of thinness and were significantly more likely to identify fatness at a thinner size than the lower SES girls in the study (Wardle *et al.* 2004). Similarly, a cross-sectional study of adult women in Canada found that women living in more affluent neighborhoods were significantly more likely to report body dissatisfaction, independent of personal affluence, than women in less affluent neighborhoods (McLaren and Gauvin 2002).

To date, Stice *et al.* (2004) have conducted the only randomized investigation of the impact of peer pressure to be thin on young women's body dissatisfaction, a potent risk factor for eating pathology (Stice 2002). The researchers randomly assigned women to a condition wherein a very thin confederate complained about how fat she felt and expressed intentions to lose weight or a control condition wherein she discussed a neutral topic. Women exposed to peer pressure to be thin reported significant increases in body dissatisfaction relative to those women in the control condition. In contrast to experimental evidence for the mediating pathways of thin-ideal internalization and social comparison in the relation between media exposure and body image and eating disturbance, this experiment found a direct relationship between peer pressure to be thin and body dissatisfaction (Stice *et al.* 2004). As these studies demonstrate, localized social climates indeed reinforce broader cultural values and norms of perform-ance and appearance. Additional studies are needed to examine the potentially interactive effects of peer-derived social pressure and comparison on dis-ordered eating.

Family influence

Family relations are another level of social influence that further reinforce cultural ideals that perpetuate eating pathology. The reinforcement may be direct, such as through explicit encouragement to diet or lose weight, or it may occur indirectly through parental modeling behaviors and attitudes. For ex-ample, among preadolescent girls, family pressure to be thin affects body dissatisfaction more than pressure from either the media or peers. In addition, parental modeling of disordered eating behaviors was associated with increased body dissatisfaction (Blowers *et al.* 2003). Other evidence suggests that parents can influence children's eating and weight problems by fostering a home environment with a high emphasis on thinness and attractiveness. In one study of college women, Davis and colleagues (2004) found that a family focus on appearance was related to weight preoccupation among those women reporting above-normal neuroticism scores. In a large sample of adolescents, Neumark-Sztainer and colleagues (2002) found that family weight norms (e.g. parental dieting or encouragement of child's weight loss) indirectly predicted unhealthy weight control behaviors through the pathway of adolescent weight-body concern. Finally, perceived pressure from family members to maintain a thin body shape–though a less potent predictor than peer pressure–was associated with increased bulimic tendencies in a sample of college women (Young *et al.* 2004). These studies strongly suggest that familial behaviors and attitudes may provide an overlapping social domain that moderates risk for disordered eating.

Teasing

Teasing or weight-related criticism/discrimination is an important pathway through which peers or family members may exert their influence on body and self-evaluation, presumably by highlighting divergence from ideal attributes and social norms (Neumark-Sztainer *et al.* 2002). Among a diverse adolescent population, weight-related teasing by peers and family members was consist-ently associated with low body satisfaction and self-esteem. Moreover, the impact of teasing on self- and body-esteem was found to be independent of adolescents' actual weight (Eisenberg *et al.* 2003). Another study identified teasing as associated with an increased drive for thinness and restricted eating among adolescent females from Bombay, India (Shroff and Thompson 2004). While numerous studies have implicated the role of weight-related teasing in disordered eating, less attention has been focused on racial teasing and dis-crimination. Among south Asian college women, a history of racial teasing was associated with disturbed eating and body image, even after controlling for distress, self-esteem and BMI (Iyer and Haslam 2003). In addition, White women with BED reported significantly higher rates of ethnic or racial discrimination than healthy comparison subjects (Striegel-Moore *et al.* 2002).

Methodologic challenges relevant to cross-ethnic and transcultural research

Several methodologic problems continue to pose serious challenges to the interpretation of research findings from transcultural studies. First, school-based recruitment is likely to be associated with Western, educational, or social influences that introduce selection bias and are difficult to ascertain and adjust for. Second, assessments are infrequently validated and checked for reliability relative to the new study population. This is likely to result in outcome misclassification that introduces bias of unknown magnitude and direction. Le Grange *et al.* (2004) describe an extraordinary illustration of outcome mis-classification in a study of Black South Africans. Moreover, Franko *et al.* (2004) have demonstrated substantive differences between White and Black ado-lescents on the factor structure of the EDI. Finally, the variation in assessments and outcomes under investigation makes cross-cultural prevalence comparison difficult.

Additional methodologic concerns apply to investigation of sociocultural risk factors for eating disorders. First, consistent definition and operationalization of possible predictors such as acculturation, westernization and modernization remain elusive. Even the concepts of race (a biologic designation) and ethnicity (cultural and self-identity designations) have been used inconsistently and interchangeably. Next, there has been incomplete appreciation of the ways in which such categories as 'Black' and 'Hispanic' may have quite distinct meanings from one continent to another and for the heterogeneity of ethnicity within these racial categories–especially among Latino populations. Third, small cell counts within various observational strata often limit the necessary statistical power for inference about differences among these populations. Finally, with several notable exceptions, qualitative research continues to be underutilized in understanding sociocultural contributions to disturbed body image and disordered eating. For example, ethnographic and narrative data from Curacao (Katzman *et al.* 2004), Fiji (Becker 2004), Belize (Anderson-Fye 2004), and Japan (Pike and Borovoy 2004) have demonstrated the cultural specificity of symptom meanings as well as effects of mass media, westerniza-tion and acculturation. These studies augment the seminal work by Lee and colleagues (2001) demonstrating the phenomenologic variation in AN across cultural contexts. They also provide a thicker description of how social pro-cesses underpin eating symptoms (*see* Lee 2004). Furthermore, incorporation of qualitative data into study design will be essential to interpreting local cultural meanings of disordered eating, understanding differential risk and suggesting situation-specific interventions.

Summary of important findings

In the past several years, epidemiologic studies have continued to provide evidence for the global distribution of eating disorders across diverse social contexts. They have also presented contradictory data on estimates of comparative prevalence across ethnic populations in the US. Specifically, the similarity of prevalence among major ethnic groups in the US has been supported by several recent large studies. Other evidence continues to support elevated risk among Native Americans and reduced risk among African-Americans. New findings have been consistent in contradicting previous data that BED may have been more prevalent among Black women than White women.

On the one hand, the emphasis on convergence of prevalence is welcome given that ethnic disparities in access to care for eating disorders have emerged as a socially and clinically important problem. Educating families, clinicians, teachers and coaches about risk of disordered eating across diverse populations may be an important means of achieving equity in access to care. On the other hand, cultural variation in moderation of etiologic pathways remains incompletely understood and underresearched. Specifically, cultural and ethnic differences in esthetic body ideals, valuation of dimensions of self-presentation, and perception that body shape or weight may mediate social mobility may all prove important effect modifiers of the relation between the thin ideal and risk for disordered eating. Clarification and improved understanding of culture-specific risk factors for disturbed body image and eating will be essential to more effective and culturally attuned interventions.

Evidence supporting the influence of mass media, peers, family and teasing on disordered eating continues to suggest modifiable risk factors for eating disorders. However, in many respects, studies supporting these influences arguably reference *psychological* rather than social processes. That is, these studies have investigated how individuals are influenced and motivated by social values and ideals. As such, the majority of studies in this area have focused on variation in social environment (e.g. in body ideals) rather than in the culturally mediated response to the environment or in broader social processes that pattern ideas, values and behaviors. Broadening of scope and multidisciplinary methodologic strategies will thus be essential to promoting an understanding of cultural mediation of risk for eating disorders. It is likely that we will glean critical data for potential interventions from both differences and similarities across ethnically and culturally diverse populations.

Clinical implications

Advances in understanding sociocultural contributions to risk for eating disorders are critical to the development of effective and culturally sensitive prevention and intervention programs. Moreover, to the extent that prevention programs are developed to moderate influences of the social environment on disordered eating, any refinement in understanding similarities and differences in etiologic pathways and resilience across diverse social populations will assist in their strategic enhancement.

Next, given the evidence that eating disorders have global distribution and *may* be approaching parity among some ethnic minority populations, ensuring broad access to treatment for eating disorders and addressing shortfalls in recognition of eating disorders across all populations appear particularly urgent. Of particular concern are some data that suggest disparities in access to care for eating disorders across socially disadvantaged populations. Relevant intervention may require public health measures that ensure broad access and train clinicians to appreciate that diverse populations are at risk for an eating disorder diagnosis.

Finally, potential public health measures to promote prevention may require broader and more imaginative remedies at a population level than patient, family, or school-based interventions. Clarification of the adverse impact of mass media on adolescent health will support efforts for social policy changes (e.g. more rigid constraints on programming) that will help to reduce risk for vulnerable populations.

Future directions in understanding sociocultural contributions to risk

Methodologic challenges to this field include confirming validity and reliability of assessments in diverse populations, eliminating potential selection biases in study participation that would result in overrepresentation of symptoms or cases among some ethnic populations (i.e. school-based recruitment), and enhancing comparability across studies by choosing like assessments and outcomes. Improved operationalization and standardized definition of concepts such as ethnicity and acculturation will be essential as well.

The early phase of cross-ethnic and cross-cultural epidemiologic research in eating disorders was motivated by an interest in identifying characteristics of the social environment that moderated risk. This research focused on cross-cultural variation of body ideals (and the ubiquitous social pressures to be slim in the emerging global culture) without much depth in exploring how social processes might modify social comparison, motivation to reshape the body, the relative valuation of appearance in self-presentation, self-determination with respect to weight, etc. Empirical support for ways in which social environment predicts risk for disordered eating requires refinement for application to more ethnically and culturally diverse populations. Additional avenues for elucidating cultural moderation of etiologic pathways include understanding of causal effects of identification with more than one cultural group, social disparities, and disenfranchisement, as well as effect modification of ethnicity on peer and family environment and teasing on eating disorders.

Corresponding author: Anne E Becker, MD, PhD, ScM, Director, Eating Disorders Clinical and Research Program, Massachusetts General Hospital–WAC 816, 15 Parkman Street, Boston, MA 02114, USA. Email: abecker@partners.org

References

References preceded by three asterisks are of particular significance. The significance is explained by a short commentary following the complete reference.

Allison KC and Park CL (2004) A prospective study of disordered eating among sorority and nonsorority women. *International Journal of Eating Disorders*, **35**: 354–8.

Alvarez D and Paredes F (2001) *Validación del Eating Disorders Inventory (EDI) en población mexicana*. Thesis for Degree in Psychology. Universidad Nacional Autónoma de México/ ENEP Iztacala, Mexico City.

Anderson-Fye EP (2004) A Coca-Cola shape: cultural change, body image, and eating disorders in San Andrés, Belize. *Culture, Medicine and Psychiatry*, **28**: 561–95.

Anderson-Fye EP and Becker AE (2003) Eating disorders across cultures. In: JK Thompson (ed.), *Handbook of Eating Disorders and Obesity*. Wiley, New Jersey, pp 565–89.

Baranowski MJ, Jorga J, Djordjevic I, Marinkovic J and Hetherington MM (2003) Evaluation of adolescent body satisfaction and associated eating disorder pathology in two communities. *European Eating Disorders Review*, **11**: 478–95.

Becker AE (2003) Eating disorders and social transition. *Primary Psychiatry*, **10**: 75–9.

Becker AE (2004) Television, disordered eating, and young women in Fiji: Negotiating body image and identity during rapid social change. *Culture, Medicine and Psychiatry*, **28**: 533–59.

Becker AE, Burwell RA, Gilman SE, Herzog DB and Hamburg P (2002) Eating behaviors and attitudes following prolonged exposure to television among ethnic Fijian adolescent girls. *British Journal of Psychiatry*, **180**: 509–14.

Becker AE, Burwell RA, Navara K and Gilman SE (2003) Binge eating and binge eating disorder in a small-scale, indigenous society: The view from Fiji. *International Journal of Eating Disorders*, **34**: 423–31.

Becker AE, Franko DL, Speck A and Herzog DB (2003) Ethnicity and differential access to care for eating disorder symptoms. *International Journal of Eating Disorders*, **33**: 205–12.

Bendall P, Hamilton M and Holden N (1991) Eating disorders in Asian girls. *British Journal of Psychiatry*, **159**: 44I.

Bennett D, Sharpe M, Freeman C and Carson A (2004) Anorexia nervosa among female secondary school students in Ghana. *British Journal of Psychiatry*, **185**: 312–7.

Bhugra D and Bhui K (2003) Eating disorders in teenagers in East London: A survey. *European Eating Disorders Review*, **11**: 46–57.

Bhugra D, Mastrogianni A, Maharajh H and Harvey S (2003) Prevalence of bulimic behaviors and eating attitudes in schoolgirls from Trinidad and Barbados. *Transcultural Psychiatry*, **40**: 409–28.

Bilukha OO and Utermohlen V (2002) Internalization of Western standards of appearance, body dissatisfaction and dieting in urban educated Ukrainian females. *European Eating Disorders Review*, **10**: 120–37.

Blowers LC, Loxton NJ, Grady-Flesser M, Occhipinti S and Dawe S (2003) The relationship between sociocultural pressure to be thin and body dissatisfaction in adolescent girls. *Eating Behaviors*, **4**: 229–44.

Bojorquez I and Unikel C (2004) Presence of disordered eating among Mexican teenage women from a semi-urban area: its relation to the cultural hypothesis. *European Eating Disorders Review*, **12**: 197–202.

Cachelin FM, Rebeck R, Veisel C and Striegel-Moore RH (2001) Barriers to treatment for eating disorders among ethnically diverse women. *International Journal of Eating Disorders*, **30(3)**: 269–78.

Cachelin FM, Weiss JW and Garbanati JA (2003) Dieting and its relationship to smoking, acculturation, and family environment in Asian and Hispanic adolescents. *Eating Disorders,* **11**: 51–61.

Davis C and Katzman M (1999) Perfection as acculturation: Psychological correlates of eating problems in Chinese male and female students living in the United States. *International Journal of Eating Disorders,* **25(1)**: 65–70.

Davis C, Shuster B, Blackmore E and Fox J (2004) Looking good—family focus on appearance and the risk for eating disorders. *International Journal of Eating Disorders,* **35**: 136–44.

Davison KK, Earnest MB and Birch LL (2002) Participation in aesthetic sports and girls' weight concerns at ages 5 and 7 years. *International Journal of Eating Disorders,* **31**: 312–17.

Edman JL and Yates A (2004) Eating disorder symptoms among Pacific Island and Caucasian women: The impact of self dissatisfaction and anger discomfort. *Journal of Mental Health,* **13(2)**: 143–60.

Eisenberg ME, Neumark-Sztainer D and Story M (2003) Associations of weight-based teasing and emotional well-being among adolescents. *Archives of Pediatric and Adolescent Medicine,* **157**: 733–8.

Evans PC (2003) 'If only I were thin like her, maybe I could be happy like her': The self-implications of associating a thin female ideal with life success. *Psychology of Women Quarterly,* **27**: 209–14.

Festinger L (1954) A theory of social comparison processes. *Human Relations,* **7**: 117–40.

Fouts G and Vaughan K (2002) Locus of control, television viewing, and eating disorder symptomatology in young females. *Journal of Adolescence,* **25**: 307–11.

Franko DL, Striegel-Moore RH, Barton BA, Schumann BC, Garner DM, Daniels SR, Schreiber GB and Crawford PB (2004) Measuring eating concerns in Black and White adolescent girls. *International Journal of Eating Disorders,* **35**: 179–89.

Freedman R, Carter MM, Sbrocco T and Gray JJ (2004) Ethnic differences in preferences for female weight and waist-to-hip ratio: A comparison of African-American and White American college and community samples. *Eating Behaviors,* **5**: 191–8.

Frisby CM (2004) Does race matter? Effects of idealised images on African American women's perceptions of body esteem. *Journal of Black Studies,* **34(3)**: 323–47.

Garner DM (1998) *Inventario de Trastornos de la Conducta Alimentaria (EDI-2).* TEA, Madrid.

Garner DM, Garfinkel PE, Schwartz D and Thompson M (1980) Cultural expectations of thinness in women. *Psychological Reports,* **47**: 483–91.

Gilbert N and Meyer C (2003) Social anxiety and social comparison: Differential links with restrictive and bulimic attitudes among nonclinical women. *Eating Behaviors,* **4**: 257–64.

Gordon KH, Perez M and Joiner TE (2002) The impact of racial stereotypes on eating disorder recognition. *International Journal of Eating Disorders,* **32(2)**: 219–24.

Groesz LM, Levine MP and Murnen SK (2002) The effect of experimental presentation of thin media images on body satisfaction: A meta-analytic review. *International Journal of Eating Disorders,* **31**: 1–16.

Halliwell E and Dittmar H (2004) Does size matter? The impact of model's body size on women's body-focused anxiety and advertising effectiveness. *Journal of Social and Clinical Psychology,* **23(1)**: 104–22.

Hargreaves D and Tiggemann M (2003a) The effects of 'thin ideal' television commercials on body dissatisfaction and schema activation during early adolescence. *Journal of Youth and Adolescence,* **32(5)**: 367–73.

Hargreaves D and Tiggemann M (2003b) Longer-term implications of responsiveness to 'thin-ideal' television: Support for a cumulative hypothesis of body image disturbance. *European Eating Disorders Review,* **11**: 465–77.

Hausenblas HA, Janelle CM, Gardner RE and Focht BC (2004) Viewing physique slides: Affective responses of women at high and low drive for thinness. *Journal of Social and Clinical Psychology*, **23(1)**: 45–60.

Hawks SR, Madanat HN, Merrill RM, Goudy MB and Miyagawa T (2003) A cross-cultural analysis of 'motivation for eating' as a potential factor in the emergence of global obesity: Japan and the United States. *Health Promotion International*, **18(2)**: 153–62.

Hermes SF and Keel PK (2003) The influence of puberty and ethnicity on awareness and internalization of the thin ideal. *International Journal of Eating Disorders*, **33**: 465–7.

Humphrey T and Ricciardelli L (2004) The development of eating pathology in Chinese-Australian women: Acculturation versus culture clash. *International Journal of Eating Disorders*, **35**: 579–88.

Iyer DS and Haslam N (2003) Body image and eating disturbance among South Asian-American women: The role of racial teasing. *International Journal of Eating Disorders*, **34**: 142–7.

Joshi R, Herman CP and Polivy J (2004) Self-enhancing effects of exposure to thin-body images. *International Journal of Eating Disorders*, **35**: 333–41.

Kaltiala-Heino R, Kautiainen S, Virtanen SM, Rimpela A and Rimpelä M (2003) Has the adolescents' weight concern increased over 20 years? *Health Behavior*, **13**: 4–10.

Katzman MA, Hermans KME, Van Hoeken D and Hoek HW (2004) Not your 'typical island woman': Anorexia nervosa is reported only in subcultures in Curacao. *Culture, Medicine and Psychiatry*, **28(4)**: 463–92.

***Keel PK and Klump KL (2003) Are eating disorders culture-bound syndromes? Implications for conceptualizing their etiology? *Psychological Bulletin*, **129(5)**: 747–69.

This extremely comprehensive literature review examines evidence for sociocultural and genetic contributions to risk for eating disorders. These authors present a novel argument that whereas AN appears to arise in the absence of a cultural valuation of thinness, cross-cultural studies do support that BN occurs exclusively in the context of Western cultural influence. They further suggest that heritability estimates for BN may show greater cross-cultural variability than heritability estimates for AN.

Lee S (1996) Reconsidering the status of anorexia nervosa as a Western culture-bound syndrome. *Social Science and Medicine*, **42**: 21–34.

***Lee S (2004) Engaging culture: an overdue task for eating disorders research. *Culture, Medicine and Psychiatry*, **28**: 617–21.

This commentary by one of the preeminent researchers in cultural mediation of eating disorders advocates greater use of ethnography in elucidating social processes underpinning eating disorders. It references his own pioneering work in describing a phenomenologically distinct presentation of AN in China–that is, one with absent fat phobia. Dr Lee's commentary is one among several by experts in the cross-cultural study of eating disorders–Richard Gordon, Roland Littlewood and Rebecca Lester–on a collection of studies on new global perspectives on body image that comprise a special issue of *Culture, Medicine and Psychiatry* and include original studies from qualitative work in Belize, Fiji, Japan, South Africa and Curacao.

Lee S, Lee AM, Ngai E, Lee D and Wing YK (2001) Rationales for food refusal in Chinese patients with anorexia nervosa. *International Journal of Eating Disorders*, **29(2)**: 224–9.

Le Grange D, Louw J, Breen A and Katzman MA (2004) The meaning of 'self-starvation' in impoverished Black adolescents in South Africa. *Culture, Medicine and Psychiatry*, **28(4)**: 439–61.

Lin LF and Kulik JA (2002) Social comparison and women's body satisfaction. *Basic and Applied Social Psychology*, **24(2)**: 115–23.

Low KG, Charanasomboon S, Brown C, Hiltunen G, Long K and Reinhalter K (2003) Internalization of the thin ideal, weight and body image concerns. *Social Behavior and Personality*, **31(1)**: 81–90.

Lynch WC, Eppers KD and Sherrod JR (2004) Eating attitudes of Native American and White female adolescents: A comparison of BMI- and age-matched groups. *Ethnicity & Health*, **9(3)**: 253–66.

McLaren L and Gauvin L (2002) Neighbourhood level versus individual level correlates of women's body dissatisfaction: Toward a multilevel understanding of the role of affluence. *Journal of Epidemiology and Community Health*, **56(3)**: 193–7.

Morrison T, Waller G, Meyer C, Burditt E, Wright F, Babbs M and Gilbert N (2003) Social comparison in the eating disorders. *Journal of Nervous and Mental Disease*, **191(8)**: 553–5.

Mumford DB, Whitehouse AM and Platts M (1991) Sociocultural correlates of eating disorders among Asian schoolgirls in Bradford. *British Journal of Psychiatry*, **158**: 222–8.

Murnen SK, Smolak L, Mills JA and Good L (2003) Thin, sexy women and strong, muscular men: Grade-school children's responses to objectified images of women and men. *Sex Roles*, **49(9/10)**: 427–37.

Nasser M (1986) Comparative study of the prevalence of abnormal eating attitudes among Arab female students of both London and Cairo universities. *Psychological Medicine*, **16**: 621–5.

Nasser M, Katzman MA and Gordon RA (2001) *Eating Disorders and Cultures in Transition*. Brunner-Routledge, East Sussex.

Neumark-Sztainer D, Falkner N, Story M, Perry C, Hannan PJ and Mulert S (2002) Weight-based teasing among adolescents: Correlations with weight status and disordered eating behaviors. *International Journal of Obesity*, **26**: 123–31.

Neumark-Sztainer D, Wall M, Story M and Perry C (2003) Correlates of unhealthy weight-control behaviors among adolescents: Implications for programs. *Health Psychology*, **22(1)**: 88–98.

Nunes MA, Barros FC, Anselmo Olinto MT, Camey S and Mari JDJ (2003) Prevalence of abnormal eating behaviors and inappropriate methods of weight control in young women from Brazil: A population-based study. *Eating and Weight Disorders*, **8**: 100–6.

O'Neill SK (2003) African American women and eating disturbances: A meta-analysis. *Journal of Black Psychology*, **29(1)**: 3–16.

Oyewumi LK and Kazarian SS (1992) Abnormal eating attitudes among a group of Nigerian youths: II. Anorexic behavior. *East African Medical Journal*, **69**: 667–9.

Perez M and Joiner TE (2003) Body image dissatisfaction and disordered eating in Black and White women. *International Journal of Eating Disorders*, **33**: 342–50.

Pike KM and Borovoy A (2004) The rise of eating disorders in Japan: Issues of culture and limitations of the model of 'westernization'. *Culture, Medicine and Psychiatry*, **28(4)**: 493–531.

Pike KM and Mizushima H (2005) The clinical presentation of Japanese women with anorexia nervosa and bulimia nervosa: A study of the eating disorders inventory-2. *International Journal of Eating Disorders*, **37(1)**: 26–31.

Presnell K, Bearman SK and Stice E (2004) Risk factors for body dissatisfaction in adolescent boys and girls: A prospective study. *International Journal of Eating Disorders*, **36**: 389–401.

Rubin LR, Fitts ML and Becker AE (2003) 'Whatever feels good in my soul': Body ethics and aesthetics among African American and Latina women. *Culture, Medicine and Psychiatry*, **27**: 49–75.

Sanchez-Johnsen L, Dymek M, Alverdy J and LeGrange D (2003) Binge eating and eating-related cognitions and behavior in ethnically diverse obese women. *Obesity Research*, **11**: 1002–9.

Schooler D, Ward LM, Merriwether A and Caruthers A (2004) Who's that girl: Television's role in the body image development of young white and black women. *Psychology of Women Quarterly*, **28**: 38–47.

***Shaw H, Ramirez L, Trost A, Randall P and Stice E (2004) Body image and eating disturbances across ethnic groups: More similarities than differences. *Psychology of Addictive Behaviors*, **18(1)**: 12–18.

This is a methodologically rigorous study that presents data that suggest that ethnic groups have reached parity in terms of eating disturbances. It utilizes a large, ethnically diverse sample, incorporates data from psychiatric interviews, and examines ethnicity as a moderator between risk factors and eating disorder outcomes.

Shroff H and Thompson JK (2004) Body image and eating disturbance in India: Media and interpersonal influences. *International Journal of Eating Disorders*, **35**: 198–203.

Stice E (2001) A prospective test of the dual-pathway model of bulimic pathology: Mediating effects of dieting and negative affect. *Journal of Abnormal Psychology*, **110(1)**: 124–35.

Stice E (2002) Risk and maintenance factors for eating pathology: A meta-analytic review. *Psychological Bulletin*, **128(5)**: 825–48.

Stice E and Shaw H (1994) Adverse effects of the media portrayed thin-ideal on women and linkages to bulimic symptomatology. *Journal of Social and Clinical Psychology*, **13**: 288–308.

***Stice E, Maxfield J and Wells T (2004) Adverse effects of social pressure to be thin on young women: An experimental investigation of the effects of 'fat talk'. *International Journal of Eating Disorders*, **34**: 108–17.

This innovative study is the only randomized experiment to assess the impact of peer pressure to be thin on body dissatisfaction and affect in college women. Participants were randomly assigned to a condition wherein an ultra-thin confederate complained about how fat she felt and voiced intentions to lose weight or a control condition wherein she discussed a neutral topic. Consistent with studies of the role of media pressures on body image, these researchers found that peer pressure to be thin also resulted in increased body dissatisfaction but not negative affect. Interestingly, however, these effects were not moderated by thin ideal internalization, body dissatisfaction, or social support. These findings suggest the importance of further research on peer influences in the perpetuation of disordered eating.

Striegel-Moore RH, Silberstein LR and Rodin J (1986) Toward an understanding of risk factors for bulimia. *American Psychologist*, **41**: 246–63.

Striegel-Moore RH, Dohm F, Pike KM, Wilfley DE and Fairburn CG (2002) Abuse, bullying, and discrimination as risk factors for binge eating disorder. *American Journal of Psychiatry*, **159**: 1902–07.

***Striegel-Moore RH, Dohm F, Kraemer HC, Taylor CB, Daniels S, Crawford P and Shreiber GB (2003) Eating disorders in White and Black women. *American Journal of Psychiatry*, **160**: 1326–31.

This study of the prevalence of AN, BN and BED in a large, prospective cohort of Black and White women challenges prior data suggesting an increased prevalence of BED among Black as compared to White women. This study's recruitment of a geographically and socio-economically diverse, community-based sample makes an important contribution to understanding of the prevalence of eating disorders among Black women.

Sypeck MF, Gray JJ and Ahrens AH (2004) No longer just a pretty face: Fashion magazines' depictions of ideal female beauty from 1959–1999. *International Journal of Eating Disorders*, **36**: 342–7.

Tareen A, Hodes M and Rangel L (2005) Non-fat-phobic anorexia nervosa in British South Asian adolescents. *International Journal of Eating Disorders*, **37(2)**: 161–5.

Thompson SH and Digsby S (2004) A preliminary survey of dieting, body dissatisfaction, and eating problems among high school cheerleaders. *Journal of School Health*, **74(3)**: 85–90.

Tiggemann M (2003) Media exposure, body dissatisfaction and disordered eating: Television and magazines are not the same! *European Eating Disorders Review*, **11**: 418–30.

Tiggemann M and Slater A (2004) Thin ideals in music television: A source of social comparison and body dissatisfaction. *International Journal of Eating Disorders*, **35**: 48–58.

Tölgyes T and Nemessury J (2004) Epidemiological studies on adverse dieting behaviors and eating disorders among young people in Hungary. *Social Psychiatry and Psychiatric Epidemiology*, **39**: 647–54.

Tong J, Miao S, Wang J, Zhang JJ, Wu HM, Li T *et al.* (2005) Five cases of male eating disorders in central China. *International Journal of Eating Disorders*, **37(1)**: 72–5.

Troop NA, Allan S, Treasure JL and Katzman M (2003) Social comparison and submissive behavior in eating disorder patients. *Psychology and Psychotherapy: Theory, Research, and Practice*, **76**: 237–49.

Tsai G, Curbow B and Heinberg L (2003) Sociocultural and developmental influences on body dissatisfaction and disordered eating attitudes and behaviors of Asian women. *Journal of Nervous and Mental Disease*, **191(5)**: 309–18.

Van den Berg P, Thompson JK, Obremski-Brandon K and Coovert M (2002) The tripartite influence model of body image and eating disturbance: A covariance structure modeling investigation testing the mediational role of appearance comparison. *Journal of Psychosomatic Research*, **53(7378)**: 1007–20.

Voracek M and Fisher ML (2002) Shapely centerfolds? Temporal changes in body measures: Trend analysis. *British Medical Journal*, **325(3)**: 1447–8.

Wardle J and Watters R (2004) Sociocultural influences on attitudes to weight and eating: Results of a natural experiment. *International Journal of Eating Disorders*, **35**: 589–96.

Wardle J, Robb KA, Johnson F, Griffith J, Brunner E, Power C and Tovèe M (2004) Socioeconomic variation in attitudes to eating and weight in female adolescents. *Health Psychology*, **23(3)**: 275–82.

Wesch SL (2004) *Factors related to appearance satisfaction among women native to the Mountain Ok area of Papua New Guinea* (unpublished doctoral dissertation). American University, Washington DC.

White MA, Kohlmaier JR, Varnado-Sullivan P and Williamson DA (2003) Racial/ethnic differences in weight concerns: Protective and risk factors for the development of eating disorders and obesity among adolescent females. *Eating and Weight Disorders*, **8**: 20–5.

Yang CJ, Gray P and Pope HG (2005) Male body image in Taiwan versus the West: Yanggang Zhiqi meets the Adonis complex. *American Journal of Psychiatry*, **162(2)**: 263–9.

Young EA, Clopton JR and Bleckley MK (2004) Perfectionism, low self-esteem, and family factors as predictors of bulimic behavior. *Eating Behaviors*, **5**: 273–83.

4

Epidemiology of eating disorders: an update

Ruth H Striegel-Moore, Debra L Franko and Emily L Ach

Abstract

Objectives of review. Epidemiological studies of eating disorders published between 2003 and 2005 were reviewed to examine the distribution of anorexia nervosa (AN), bulimia nervosa (BN) and binge-eating disorder (BED) in the population.

Summary of recent findings. In females, the reported point prevalence estimates of AN ranged from 0 to 1.5 while estimates of BN ranged from 0.37 to 3.0. Females' lifetime prevalence estimates for AN ranged from 0.6 to 4.0 and from 1.2 to 5.9 for BN. AN and BN were rare among males. For BED, point prevalence ranged from 0.4 to 0.7 and lifetime estimates ranged from 0.6 to 2.7. Methodological limitations of studies include the variability in instruments used to diagnose eating disorders and the lack of an agreed definition for Eating Disorders, Not Otherwise Specified (EDNOS).

Future directions. Epidemiological data from a nationally representative sample in the US are needed. Future research should examine the prevalence of EDNOS, pending the development of a universal definition of this disorder.

Introduction

Epidemiology concerns itself with the study of the distribution of diseases in the population and the factors that explain risk for the development or clinical course of disorders. Underlying epidemiological research is the assumption that diseases do not occur at random; rather, it is assumed that some individuals are more likely to fall ill than others. Epidemiological studies seek to uncover factors that explain differential risk for the development of the disorder under investigation. It is well established that risk for experiencing health or mental health problems varies by gender, race/ethnicity, age and socioeconomic status. For example, in the case of eating disorders, girls or women are more likely than boys or men to experience eating disorder symptoms or syndromes, and the complex reasons for this gender disparity have been the subject of extensive theoretical and empirical research (Rodin *et al.* 1985c; Jacobi *et al.* 2004).

Studies of the prevalence and incidence of eating disorders seek to identify the number of affected individuals in a given time period ('prevalence') and new-onset or newly identified cases ('incidence'); this paper focuses solely on prevalence because no new studies of incidence have been reported. Studies seeking to identify risk factors for the development of an eating disorder beyond the basic demographic characteristics are discussed by Jacobi (2005) and will not be covered here. The present paper is organized into three major sections: we first review the literature, highlighting key findings and methodological considerations; next we consider the clinical or practical implications of the findings; and then conclude with suggestions for future research.

To identify relevant articles, we conducted a Medline search that was restricted to 'English language in years 2003–2005' and used the search terms 'epidemiology', 'incidence', or 'prevalence' in combination with 'anorexia nervosa', 'bulimia nervosa', or 'eating disorders' in the title. Because of the apparent liberal use of the terms 'prevalence' or 'incidence', this strategy yielded well over 100 citations. From this list, citations were extracted that described studies (a) involving community samples (thereby excluding any study using patient samples); or (b) reporting on special populations that have received no or relatively limited attention in previous reviews (e.g. individuals with type I diabetes); and (c) using an interview for determining case status (thus eliminating any study that based diagnosis solely on self-report questionnaires). The latter criterion was employed because experts agree that ascertainment of case status based exclusively on self-report questionnaire data is too inaccurate (typically generating many false–positive cases) to provide valid prevalence estimates (Fairburn and Beglin 1990; Lewinsohn *et al.* 2002; Hoek and van Hoeken 2003).

Representativeness of study samples is a fundamental requirement in epidemiological studies. Given the complete lack of such data in the United States (US) (and in many other countries) concerning eating disorders, this review includes papers that involve non-representative samples.

Review of the literature

Our paper seeks to update three relevant recently published narrative reviews; these earlier reviews provide an important launching point for the present review, which is restricted to publications dated 2003 or later.

Recent reviews of prevalence studies

The first review (Hoek and van Hoeken 2003) reported on studies of the prevalence and incidence of eating disorders through 2002. The authors concluded that anorexia nervosa (AN) had an average prevalence of 0.3% in community samples of young females and that, based on referral rates to inpatient facilities, the number of newly detected ('incidence') cases likely had increased over the past century until the 1970s. The authors found no studies reporting the incidence of bulimia nervosa (BN). Average prevalence of BN and of binge-eating disorder (BED) in community samples were both estimated as approximately 1%. A robust finding is that females are far more likely than males and adults are more likely than adolescents to experience an eating disorder.

The first author of the present paper wrote the section on epidemiology for the eating disorder chapter of the Annenberg Commission on Adolescent Mental Health (Commission on Adolescent Eating Disorders, in press). Conclusions from the review of studies of the prevalence or incidence data for AN, BN and their spectrum variants in adolescents (i.e. children aged 12 to 18 years) were that most studies recruited samples of convenience and lacked adequate sample sizes, minority populations were seriously under-represented and methodologies varied widely across studies. Given the prevalence estimates reported in previous studies, it is apparent that large samples are needed to find any cases and examine even the most commonly studied epidemiological variables such as gender or ethnicity. Indeed, even in samples exceeding 1000 girls, some studies have not identified a single girl with past or current AN (Johnson-Sabine et al. 1988). Nevertheless, because of the rather preliminary stage of epidemiological research among adolescent samples in particular, for the present review studies were included even if they were based on relatively small or select samples.

Makino et al. (2004) reviewed studies of the prevalence and self-reported symptoms of eating disorders in Western and non-Western countries. They expressed similar methodological concerns noted in the aforementioned reviews, but added that in studies of non-Western populations, survey instruments were not evaluated to determine cultural appropriateness in the target populations. The authors concluded that abnormal eating attitudes have been increasing in non-Western countries.

Prevalence studies of eating disorders

Overview

In all, 13 studies have been published since 2003 and provided interview-based information about the prevalence of full syndrome AN and BN and, in some instances, BED. The key methodological features of these studies are shown in Table 4.1 for studies that employed a two-stage case finding procedure and Table 4.2 for studies where all participants were assessed for a possible diagnosis of an eating disorder.

Methodological considerations

Ideally, an epidemiological study recruits a representative population sample, yet few such studies were found. The tables show the country where a study was conducted and provide brief information about the sampling frame. Sample sizes are reported next, indicating whenever possible gender of partici-pants and, in one instance (Striegel-Moore et al. 2003), race. Participation rate is an important indicator of possible sampling biases; where available, along with the sample size, participation rates are reported for the screening stage (see Table 4.1) and the interview stage (see Tables 4.1 and 4.2). Most studies used the two-stage screening rather than interviewing a complete population sample. It is relatively inexpensive to survey participants with self-report questionnaires; the expensive interview method typically is reserved for those participants whose self-report answers suggest presence of an eating disorder. Critically important, however, is that participation is high at each assessment stage and that the screening instrument is sufficiently sensitive: in an uncommon dis-order, missing even a few cases because of an insufficiently sensitive screening questionnaire will result in a considerable underestimation of the true preva-lence of the disorder. Although some of the studies described in Table 4.1 reported both current and lifetime disorders, authors tend not to discuss the limitation of using a self-report questionnaire to identify eating disorders in participants who at the time of the screening are no longer symptomatic. Also, not all screening questionnaires were specifically designed for detecting eating disorders. For example, the otherwise methodologically rigorous study reported by F Jacobi and colleagues (2004) sought to identify 12-month and lifetime prevalence of major mental disorders in a nationally representative sample of German adults and used an initial survey that screened broadly for psychopathology. This ap-proach may have resulted in an underestimation of eating disorder prevalence. Even questionnaires that were developed specifically for measuring eating pathology may not yield adequate estimates for specific eating disorders.

In a few studies, the assessment of all participants was based on a complete diagnostic interview (see Table 4.2). Typically, these studies determined eating disorder diagnosis in the context of a broader assessment of psychiatric disorders rather than being focused specifically on eating disorders. When participants are not recruited specifically for a study of eating disorders, participation rates

Table 4.1 Two-stage studies of the prevalence of anorexia nervosa (AN) and bulimia nervosa (BN) in community samples of female (F) and male (M) adolescents

Study	Country (city or state)	Sample*	Age (years)	Sample size (response rate in %)	Screening**/interview (response rate in %)	AN P	AN L	BN P	BN L	BED P	BED L
Patton et al. (2003)	Australia	1	14–15	982 F	BET CIS-R	0 –	1.8 –	N/A –	1.2 –	– –	–
Rojo et al. (2003)	Spain	2	12–18	544 F/M	EAT-40 Interview (96.4)	F.45 M 0	– –	F .41 M 0	– –	.41	(gender unknown)
Striegel-Moore et al. (2003)	United States	3	21.3 F (white) 21.5 F (black)	985 F (white) (84.5) 1061 F (black) (87.5)	Mini EDE/EDE (97)	– –	1.5 (white) 0 (black)	– –	2.3 (white) .4 (black)	– –	2.7 (white) 1.4 (black)
Grylli et al. (2004)	Austria	4	14.1 (mean)	F 96 (79.3) M 103	EAT-26 EDI-2	0.0	–	2.1	–	–	–
Jacobi F et al. (2004)	Germany	5	18–65	4181 F/M (87.6)	CID-I/CID-S	F .5 & M .2 for 'any eating disorder within a 12-month period' F 1.3 & M .3 for 'lifetime prevalence of any eating disorder'					

Table 4.1   Continued

Study	Country (city or state)	Subjects		Prevalence rates (%)		AN		BN		BED	
		Sample*	Age (years)	Sample size (response rate in %)	Screening**/interview (response rate in %)	P	L	P	L	P	L
Sundot-Borgen & Torstveit (2004)	Norway	5, 6	F 24.7 comparison (C) F 21.4 athletes (A) M 25.2 (C) M 23.2 (A)	F 574 (C) (78) F 582 (A) (93) M 629 (C) (72) M 687 (A) (76)	EDI EDE (86–95)	F .17 (C) F 2.0 (A) M .16 (C) M 0.0 (A)	–	F 3.0 (C) F 2.0 (A) M .16 (C) M 3.0 (A)	–	–	–
Tolgyes et al. (2004)	Hungary	7	10–29	F 322 M 248	BITE/EAT Interview (16.6)	F 0 M 0	–	F .39 M 0	–	–	–
Cotrufo et al. (2005)	Italy	2	17–20	259 F (100)	EDI-2 Interview (94)	0.0	–	.77	–	.77	–

*1, secondary school students including public, private, and parochial schools; 2, regionally representative sample; 3, community sample; 4, patients with type I diabetes; 5, national probability sample; 6, entire population of Norwegian elite athletes, including public, private, and parochial schools; 7, mixed sample of high school and university students; 8, entire enrollment of grades 9 through 12 in a single New Jersey county; 9, twin sample (both twins included); 10, biological mothers of twins in study population (9)

**BET, Branched Eating Disorders Test; CIS-R, Clinical Interview Schedule-revised; EAT, Eating Attitudes Test; EDE-S, Eating Disorder Examination, Screening Version; BITE, Bulimia Investigatory Test, Edinburgh; CID-S, Composite International Diagnostic Survey; CIDI-I, Composite International Diagnostic Interview; EDI, Eating Disorder Inventory; SCID, Structured Clinical Interview for DSM-IIIR; MEDE, McKnight Eating Disorder Examination; DAWBA, Development and Well Being Assessment; DIMD, short version, Diagnostic Interview for Mental Disorders-short version.

Table 4.2 Single-stage studies of the prevalence of anorexia nervosa (AN), bulimia nervosa (BN) and binge-eating disorder (BED) in samples of female (F) and male (M) adolescents

Study	Country (city or state)	Subjects		Prevalence rates (%)		AN		BN		BED	
		Sample*	Age (years)	Sample size (response rate in %)	Screening**/ interview (response rate in %)	P	L	P	L	P	L
Emerson (2003)	Great Britain	2	5–15	10,438 F/M	DAWBA	F /M 0.1–0.4 (current eating disorder)					
Favaro et al. (2003)	Italy	2	18–25	934 F	SCID	–	F 2.0	–	F 4.6	–	F .6
McKnight Investigators (2003)	United States	8	11–14	1103 F	MEDE	F 0.0	–	–	F 0.37	–	–
Petrak et al. (2003)	Germany	4	17–40	313 (Type 1) 2046 (comparison)	DIMD-short (90.2)	0 (Type 1) 0 (comparison)	–	1.0 (Type 1) <.01 (comparison)	–	–	–
Von Ranson et al. (2003)	United States	9 10	17.5 44.2	620 F 310 F	SCID (90.7) SCID (90.2)	– –	F 4.0 F .6	– –	F 4.2 F 5.9	– –	– –

*1, secondary school students including public, private, and parochial schools; 2, regionally representative sample; 3, community sample; 4, patients with type I diabetes; 5, national probability sample; 6, entire population of Norwegian elite athletes including public, private, and parochial schools; 7, mixed sample of high school and university students; 8, entire enrollment of grades 9 through 12 in a single New Jersey county; 9, twin sample (both twins included); 10, biological mothers of twins in study population (9)

**BET, Branched Eating Disorders Test; CIS-R, Clinical Interview Schedule-revised; EAT, Eating Attitudes Test; EDE-S, Eating Disorder Examination, Screening Version; BITE, Bulimia Investigatory Test, Edinburgh; CID-S, Composite International Diagnostic Survey; CIDI-I, Composite International Diagnostic Interview; EDI, Eating Disorder Inventory; SCID, Structured Clinical Interview for DSM-IIIR; MEDE, McKnight Eating Disorder Examination; DAWBA, Development and Well Being Assessment; DIMD, short version, Diagnostic Interview for Mental Disorders-short version.

likely are unaffected by the participants' attitudes about eating disorders (e.g. wanting to avoid detection of one's eating disorder). Also, gathering diagnostic information in one step eliminates loss of data due to attrition between the screening and the diagnostic stage. Finally, this approach eliminates the problems arising from delays between the two assessments: typically, most screens measure only current eating symptoms and the longer the delay between first and second assessment, the lower the correlation between the two assessments. Related, because screens typically focus on current symptoms, one-step assessment studies are better suited for establishing lifetime prevalence.

These strengths notwithstanding, there also are potential limitations. In an effort to minimize time burden, typically these interviews employ a 'branched' approach to diagnostic assessment. Unless the participant answers 'yes' to the initial question (e.g. voluntary efforts to achieve minimal low weight in the case of AN; recurrent binge eating in the case of BN or BED), no further information is gathered about the disorder. It is unclear whether in adolescents, where the clinical presentation of eating disorders may be less prototypical than among adults, this approach results in a higher number of missed cases (false negatives) than would be the case in adult samples.

Previous studies have reported conflicting findings about biases in epidemiological studies. Although a recent paper by Mond et al. (2004) found no differences between those who responded initially to the second-stage interview and those who required several reminders, less clear was whether those who initially refused any participation in this prevalence study were different from participants who agreed to participate. It is possible that such study refusers may include individuals with eating disorders who were trying to evade detection. There may be additional confounders in non-participants that are not well understood (e.g. lack of time or interest). Issues related to how participants are recruited for epidemiological studies should be considered with regard to incentive, mode of contact, and representativeness of sample (Edwards et al. 2002).

Because the quality of the assessment is critically important for arriving at reliable prevalence estimates, the tables list the screening questionnaire (Table 4.1) and diagnostic interview (Tables 4.1 and 4.2) used for determining case status. All studies defined case status using the criteria articulated in the fourth edition of the *Diagnostic and Statistical Manual of Mental Disorders* (American Psychiatric Association 1994). BED was introduced in DSM-IV as an example of an EDNOS and a provisional diagnosis in need of further study. Although BED has attracted wide research attention in the US (an entire 2003 issue of the *International Journal of Eating Disorders* has been devoted to BED), the proposal of a new disorder (BED) has not been as well received in Europe (Fairburn and Beglin 1990). This may explain why only a couple of the studies reported prevalence information for BED and both used US samples (Striegel-Moore et al. 2003; McKnight Investigators 2003).

Some studies only reported 'point prevalence' or 'lifetime' estimates, and a few studies reported both point prevalence and lifetime estimates. The timeframes used for determining point prevalence varied, including three months (McKnight Investigators 2003), 12 months (F Jacobi et al. 2004), or 'current' (defined as at the time of the diagnostic interview) (Emerson 2003; Rojo et al.

2003; Sundgot-Borgen and Torstveit 2004; Tolgyes and Nemessury 2004; Cotrufo *et al.* 2005). Furthermore, 'lifetime prevalence' is a problematic term given that some participants may have not yet passed through the period of maximum risk for developing an eating disorder. As used in the present studies lifetime prevalence refers to the number of individuals (out of all individuals sampled) who 'ever' met criteria for an eating disorder.

Key findings

Most studies were conducted in European countries; only three examined US samples (Striegel-Moore *et al.* 2003; McKnight Investigators 2003; von Ranson *et al.* 2003). There were no studies in Africa, Asia, or South America, possibly due to our language restriction in identifying studies. Only one study (conducted in the US) examined ethnic differences in prevalence of eating disorders. Specifically Striegel-Moore and colleagues (2003) found considerably fewer cases of BN and BED in their sample of black women, relative to white women. They cautioned, however, that because of the young age of their sample (mean 21 years), their study should not be interpreted as supporting the view that black women are less likely than white women to develop eating disorders involving binge eating: the black women had a significantly later age of onset of binge eating compared to the white women.

Previous reviews found that the Eating Attitudes Test (EAT) (Garner and Garfinkel 1979) was the most commonly used screening instrument for detection of AN. Its wide use is consistent with reports that the EAT has excellent psychometric properties and is available in numerous languages (Garfinkel and Newman 2001). Jacobi, Abscal and Taylor recommended the Bulimia Test-Revised (Smith and Thelen 1984) or the Bulimia Investigatory Test (Henderson and Freeman 1987) for studies of BN or BED. The studies reviewed here employed a variety of screening instruments, making comparisons across studies difficult.

There also was little uniformity regarding the diagnostic interviews that were used to confirm case status. Among the two-stage assessment studies, only four (Patton *et al.* 2003; Striegel-Moore *et al.* 2003; F Jacobi *et al.* 2004; Sundgot-Borgen and Torstveit 2004) utilized a standardized diagnostic interview. All but one (Emerson 2003) of the one-step assessment studies used standardized psychiatric interviews, albeit each study using a different interview. Across all studies, only three employed the Eating Disorder Examination (Fairburn and Cooper 1993) for confirming case status, even though it is widely regarded as the best interview for characterizing fully eating disorder pathology.

The studies varied considerably in the size and age composition of the samples. High participation rates at the screening stage was achieved in studies of school-based samples, especially when only a single school was involved (rather than multiple schools), and tended to be lower when the geographic scope of the study was broad (e.g. capturing a representative sample of an entire state or country). Participation rates at the stage-two interview were also quite high in several of the studies, with the exception of the study by Tolgyes and

Nemessury (2004), where the interview response rate was only 16.6%. These various methodological differences make comparisons across studies difficult.

With one exception (F Jacobi *et al.* 2004) the prevalence estimates reported in the tables represent the unweighted number of individuals in a study population who met case criteria relative to all participants included in the study.

Full syndrome AN

Across the studies listed in Tables 4.1 and 4.2, full syndrome current AN was found to be relatively rare among females, with reported prevalence estimates ranging from 0 to 1.5%. The prevalence for males ranged from 0 (Patton *et al.* 2003; Rojo *et al.* 2003; Tolgyes and Nemessury 2004) to 0.16% (Sundgot-Borgen and Torstveit 2004). The considerable variations in methodology make it difficult to discern a clear trend concerning the prevalence of AN in girls and young women, but the estimates are generally consistent with earlier studies. It bears noting that two studies where no girls were identified with current AN included relatively young samples (ages 11–16 years in McKnight Investigators 2003; ages 14–15 in Patton *et al.* 2003).

Only six studies provided lifetime estimates and, of these studies, two (Emerson 2003; F Jacobi *et al.* 2004) reported lifetime prevalence of 'any eating disorder' without further diagnostic distinction. Three of the remaining studies reported fairly comparable estimates of AN, 1.5 and 2.0 (Favaro *et al.* 2003; Striegel-Moore *et al.* 2003). In contrast, the fourth study reported a low estimate of 0.6% among women (median age 44.2 years) and a high estimate of 4% for adolescent twin girls (mean age 17.5 years (von Ranson *et al.* 2003)). This study applied a liberal definition of AN, however, which may account for the large case number.

In the two studies that examined lifetime prevalence for AN in males, no cases were found (Rojo *et al.* 2003; Tolgyes and Nemessury 2004). Based on case series of patients presenting for treatment (Carlat and Camargo 1991; Carlat *et al.* 1997; Striegel-Moore *et al.* 1999) it is clear that some men do develop full syndrome AN, yet neither of these studies was powered sufficiently to provide an interpretable estimate of the true prevalence (point or lifetime) in males.

Full syndrome BN

Reported prevalence estimates of current BN in females were similar across studies, 0.37–0.77, with one exception, 3.0 (Sundgot-Borgen and Torstveit 2004). It is not obvious why BN was more common in the Norwegian study except perhaps that the sample was relatively older (mean age 24.7 years). Of the three studies that included males and assessed specifically for BN, only one found any current male cases (0.16) and this again was the Norwegian sample, for which the mean age was 25.2 years. It appears that studies with relatively higher point prevalence estimates tended to include older participants.

Five studies reported on the number of girls that had 'ever' met criteria for BN prevalence ranged from a low of 1.2% (Patton *et al.* 2003) to a high of 5.9% (von

Ranson *et al.* 2003). The latter study recruited a relatively older sample (mean age = 44.2) and employed a quite liberal definition of BN. These factors may explain the relatively high lifetime prevalence estimates. No study examined lifetime prevalence of BN in males, but the point prevalence estimates suggest that lifetime prevalence is quite low.

Partial syndrome AN and BN

Because very few studies provided data about partial syndromes, we did not review specifically for subthreshold or partial syndrome prevalence estimates. Previous studies have indicated that partial syndromes generally are more common than full syndromes (Commission on Adolescent Eating Disorders, in press). The lack of a systematic definition of partial syndromes makes it impossible to draw any conclusions about the prevalence of spectrum disorders. Uniform definitions of partial syndrome AN and BN are needed.

Prevalence of BED

Three studies reported specifically on the prevalence of current BED (defined mutually exclusively from BN). The McKnight Investigators (2003) found that 0.59% of the 11–14-year-old girls met three-month point prevalence criteria for BED. Rojo (2003) reported 0.41% and Cotrufo *et al.* (2005) 0.77%. Two studies provided lifetime prevalence estimates. Favaro *et al.* (2003) reported lifetime prevalence to be 0.6 in a sample of 18–25-year-olds and Striegel-Moore *et al.* (2003) found that estimates varied by race (2.7 for white women and 1.4 for black women). In clinical samples, onset of BED (as determined by retrospective report) has been described to occur later than BN onset (Wilfley *et al.* 2000) and there are some indications from non-representative community samples that in adults BED is more prevalent than BN (Spitzer *et al.* 1993, 2000). Thus it is possible that the relatively low prevalence estimates reflect the relatively young age of these samples.

Studies of special populations

Two studies examining the prevalence of eating disorders in individuals with diabetes were published in the past two years. In a sample of 313 consecutive adult inpatients (ages 17–40) with new-onset type I diabetes, all of whom were interviewed with the Diagnostic Interview for Mental Disorders, no cases of AN and three cases of BN (0.9%) were found (Petrak *et al.* 2003). Grylli *et al.* (2004) examined 199 adolescents with type I diabetes (mean age 14.1 years) using a two-stage screening process that included the EAT and EDI-2 in stage one followed by the EDE interview for diagnostic assessment purposes for those who scored above the cutoff on the EAT. Overall, 11.5% of females and 0% of males met diagnostic criteria for eating disorders; however, no one met criteria for AN. All cases had either BN or EDNOS. These numbers did not differ significantly from the nationally representative sample of 2046 individuals used as a comparison group by Petrak *et al.* (2003) where just one case of AN and one case of BN were found. It appears that with type I diabetes, adolescents may be at increased risk for the development of BN, but not AN.

Clinical/practical implications

Several clinical implications follow from results of prevalence studies. Because full syndrome eating disorders are a relatively low frequency occurrence, yet one that has potential major health implications, frontline providers, including primary care providers and school personnel, need to be better trained to detect cases. Currently medical schools provide little training in diagnosing eating disorders and middle or high schools are more likely to put resources toward recognition of substance abuse than eating disorders. School-based screening for eating disorders would be an important step in this direction.

For AN, case definition needs to be expanded, as the current method of detecting cases on the basis of low weight (e.g. a symptom by definition denied by the sufferer) makes it likely that cases are being missed. Experts have expressed concern that the data regarding prevalence of eating disorders in adolescents are misleading because the strict diagnostic criteria do not permit diagnosis of AN or BN among adolescents who evidence the core features of these disorders, yet have not yet developed the requisite severity or duration of the symptoms (Commission on Adolescent Eating Disorders, 2005). Examination of the prevalence of behavioral eating disorder symptoms, therefore, is indicated. These symptoms may represent the first signs of the development of a full syndrome disorder and data on their prevalence thus give an indication of the size of the 'at risk' group. Furthermore, some of the symptoms have clinical significance in their own right. For example, recurrent binge eating is associated with elevated body mass index (BMI) and may be a risk factor for obesity (Fairburn *et al.* 2000). Severe dieting has been shown to be associated with psychiatric symptoms such as depression or with other health-damaging behaviors such as smoking or use of illicit substances (Middleman *et al.* 1998).

Finally, large and nationally representative epidemiological studies are needed so that government agencies and policymakers have better information for resource allocation and service planning. Recent data suggest that many of those with eating disorders do not seek treatment, or do so years after onset, suggesting the need for outreach and screening (Striegel-Moore 2005). Pediatricians or general practitioners should be encouraged to screen for eating disorders during routine medical checkups. School-based interventions might be a useful means by which to provide help to those in need.

Future research

Research is needed to address various methodological limitations found in the literature. First and foremost is the need for a prevalence study with a nationally representative sample in the US. The absence of such an epidemiologic study in the US is a glaring gap in the knowledge base of these serious disorders. Although such studies have been conducted in several European and Australian cities, the true prevalence of eating disorders in the US is not currently known. Second, prevalence data indicate that the number of individuals meeting DSM-IV diagnostic criteria for AN and BN is exceeded by those who meet partial diagnoses (Commission on Adolescent Eating Disorders, in press). Yet, there is no clear definition of partial or spectrum syndrome for eating disorders. Third, a lack of uniform instrument for measuring eating disorder symptoms currently plagues the epidemiological literature. Fourth, few studies have examined both lifetime and point prevalence of eating disorders, and even fewer provide incidence information, resulting in little information about how many new cases of eating disorders can be expected in a given year. Fifth, although studies in clinical settings find that EDNOS is more common than cases of AN or BN, there are no prevalence studies of EDNOS published to date. Before such needed studies can be done, an agreed definition of EDNOS will be necessary. Sixth, very little information has been gathered to date regarding the prevalence of eating disorders in 'special populations', meaning those for whom eating disorders are known to be not as common, but certainly do exist. Examples of such groups include individuals with cognitive impairment, men, and children. For each of these groups well-designed epidemiological studies are lacking. Finally, the prevalence of clinically significant behavioral symptoms, such as binge eating and night eating, would be of interest as they relate to clinical syndromes of BN and BED.

Conclusions

Prevalence estimates from epidemiological studies conducted between 2003 and 2005 are generally consistent with earlier reports and indicate a higher prevalence of AN and BN among adult samples compared to adolescent samples, and very low prevalence of either disorder among males. The prevalence of eating disorders in the US is not known at this time due to the lack of studies using nationally representative samples. Finally, universal definitions of both partial syndromes and EDNOS will be necessary to facilitate future prevalence studies.

Corresponding author: Dr Ruth H Striegel-Moore, Department of Psychology, Wesleyan University, 207 High Street, Middletown, CT 06459, USA. Email: rstriegel@wesleyan.edu

References

References included from the targeted review years are preceded by one asterisk. References preceded by three asterisks are of particular significance. The significance is explained by a short commentary following the complete reference.

American Psychiatric Association (1994) *Diagnostic and Statistical Manual of Mental Disorders* (4e). American Psychiatric Publishing Inc, Washington DC.

Carlat DJ and Camargo CA Jr (1991) Review of bulimia nervosa in males. *Am J Psychiatry*, **148(7)**: 831–43.

Carlat DJ, Camargo CA Jr and Herzog DB (1997) Eating disorders in males: a report on 135 patients. *Am J Psychiatry*, **154(8)**: 1127–32.

*Commission on Adolescent Eating Disorders (in press) Defining eating disorders. In: DL Evans, EB Foa, RE Gur *et al.* (eds), *Treating and Preventing Adolescent Mental Health Disorders: what we know and what we don't know*. Oxford University Press, New York.

*Cotrufo P, Gnisci A and Caputo I (2005) Brief report: psychological characteristics of less severe forms of eating disorders: an epidemiological study among 259 female adolescents. *J Adolesc*, **28(1)**: 147–54.

Edwards P, Roberts I, Clarke M *et al.* (2002) Increasing response rates to postal questionnaires: systematic review. *BMJ*, **324**: 1183–5.

*Emerson E (2003) Prevalence of psychiatric disorders in children and adolescents with and without intellectual disability. *J Intellect Disabil Res*, **47(Pt 1)**: 51–8.

Fairburn CG and Beglin SJ (1990) Studies of the epidemiology of bulimia nervosa. *Am J Psychiatry*, **147(4)**: 401–8.

Fairburn CG and Cooper Z (1993) The Eating Disorder Examination (12e). In: CG Fairburn and GT Wilson (eds), *Binge Eating: nature, assessment, and treatment*. Guilford Press, New York, pp 317–60.

Fairburn CG, Cooper Z, Doll HA, Norman P and O'Connor M (2000) The natural course of bulimia nervosa and binge eating disorder in young women. *Arch Gen Psychiatry*, **57(7)**: 659–65.

***Favaro A, Ferrara S and Santonastaso P (2003) The spectrum of eating disorders in young women: a prevalence study in a general population sample. *Psychosom Med*, **65(4)**: 701–08.
A community-based Italian study in which the authors conducted interviews with all 934 young adult women (ages 18–25) residing in both urban and suburban areas of a large city. The authors examined both DSM-IV and partial and subthreshold eating disorders and reported prevalence estimates for anorexia nervosa, bulimia nervosa, and binge-eating disorder.

Garfinkel PE and Newman A (2001) The eating attitudes test: twenty-five years later. *Eat Weight Disord*, **6(1)**: 1–24.

Garner DM and Garfinkel PE (1979) The Eating Attitudes Test: an index of the symptoms of anorexia nervosa. *Psychol Med*, **9(2)**: 273–9.

Grylli V, Hafferl-Gattermayer A, Schober E and Karwautz A (2004) Prevalence and clinical manifestations of eating disorders in Austrian adolescents with type-1 diabetes. *Wien Klin Wochenschr*, **116(7–8)**: 230–4.

Henderson M and Freeman CP (1987) A self-rating scale for bulimia. The 'BITE'. *Br J Psychiatry*, **150**: 18–24.

*Hoek HW and van Hoeken D (2003) Review of the prevalence and incidence of eating disorders. *Int J Eat Disord*, **34**: 383–96.

Jacobi C (2005) Psychosocial risk factors for eating disorders. In: S Wonderlich, J Mitchell, M de Zwaan and H Steiger (eds), *Eating Disorders Review Part 1*. Radcliffe Publishing Ltd, Oxford, pp 59–86.

Jacobi C, Hayward C, de Zwaan M, Kraemer HC and Agras WS (2004) Coming to terms with risk factors for eating disorders: application of risk terminology and suggestions for a general taxonomy. *Psychol Bull*, **130(1)**: 19–65.

***Jacobi F, Wittchen HU, Holting C *et al.* (2004) Prevalence, co-morbidity and correlates of mental disorders in the general population: results from the German Health Interview and Examination Survey (GHS). *Psychol Med*, **34(4)**: 597–611.

The first government mandated nationwide study to examine both medical and mental disorders in 4181 adults (ages 18–65) conducted in Germany. Although diagnostic groupings for eating disorders were collapsed into one 'any eating disorder' category, prevalence estimates were obtained for the past four weeks, the previous 12 months, and lifetime history, providing a snapshot of prevalence rates at three different timeframes.

Johnson-Sabine E, Wood K, Patton G, Mann A and Wakeling A (1988) Abnormal eating attitudes in London schoolgirls–a prospective epidemiological study: factors associated with abnormal response on screening questionnaires. *Psychol Med*, **18(3)**: 615–22.

Lewinsohn PM, Seeley JR, Moerk KC and Striegel-Moore RH (2002) Gender differences in eating disorder symptoms in young adults. *Int J Eat Disord*, **32(4)**: 426–40.

*Makino M, Tsuboi K and Dennerstein L (2004) Prevalence of eating disorders: a comparison of Western and non-Western countries. *Medscape General Medicine*, **6(3)**: 49.

*McKnight Investigators (2003) Risk factors for the onset of eating disorders in adolescent girls: results of the McKnight longitudinal risk factor study. *Am J Psychiatry*, **160(2)**: 248–54.

Middleman AB, Vazquez I and Durant RH (1998) Eating patterns, physical activity and attempts to change weight among adolescents. *J Adolescent Health*, **22**: 37–42.

Mond JM, Rodgers B, Hay PJ, Owen C and Beumont PJ (2004) Nonresponse bias in a general population survey of eating-disordered behavior. *Int J Eat Disord*, **36(1)**: 89–98.

***Patton GC, Coffey C and Sawyer SM (2003) The outcome of adolescent eating disorders: findings from the Victorian Adolescent Health Cohort Study. *Eur Child Adolesc Psychiatry*, **12 Suppl 1**: I25–29.

This Australian school-based study was conducted with 932 adolescent girls over a six-year period (initial ages 14–15). Both partial and full syndrome disorders were documented and the longitudinal data permitted examination of the stability of eating disorders over time as well as health outcomes in young adulthood (e.g. depression, substance use).

*Petrak F, Hardt J, Wittchen HU *et al.* (2003) Prevalence of psychiatric disorders in an onset cohort of adults with type 1 diabetes. *Diabetes Metab Res Rev*, **19(3)**: 216–22.

Rodin J, Silberstein LR and Striegel-Moore RH (1985) Women and weight: a normative discontent. In: TB Sonderegger (ed), *Nebraska Symposium on Motivation, 1984: psychology and gender*. University of Nebraska, Lincoln, pp 267–308.

***Rojo L, Livianos L, Conesa L *et al.* (2003) Epidemiology and risk factors of eating disorders: a two-stage epidemiologic study in a Spanish population aged 12–18 years. *Int J Eat Disord*, **34(3)**: 281–91.

This is the first two-stage epidemiological study to investigate risk factors and assess prevalence rates in Spain. Interviews with 544 male and female participants (ages 12–18) included assessment of both full syndrome and partial syndromes for AN, BN, and EDNOS. Documented risk factors included having dieted in the previous year, having a friend on a diet, and psychiatric comorbidity, among others.

Smith MC and Thelen MH (1984) Development and validation of a test for bulimia. *J Consult Clin Psychol*, **52(5)**: 863–72.

Spitzer RL, Yanovski S, Wadden T *et al.* (1993) Binge eating disorder: its further validation in a multisite study. *Int J Eat Disord*, **13(2)**: 137–53.

Spitzer RL, Williams JB, Kroenke K, Hornyak R and McMurray J (2000) Validity and utility of the PRIME-MD patient health questionnaire in assessment of 3000 obstetric-gynecologic patients: the PRIME-MD Patient Health Questionnaire Obstetrics-Gynecology Study. *Am J Obstet Gynecol*, **183(3)**: 759–69.

Striegel-Moore RH (2005) Health services research in anorexia nervosa. *Int J Eat Disord*, **37**: S31–S34.

Striegel-Moore RH, Garvin V, Dohm FA and Rosenheck RA (1999) Eating disorders in a national sample of hospitalized female and male veterans: detection rates and psychiatric comorbidity. *Int J Eat Disord*, **25(4)**: 405–14.

***Striegel-Moore RH, Dohm FA, Kraemer HC, Taylor CB, Daniels S, Crawford PB *et al.* (2003) Eating disorders in white and black women. *Am J Psychiatry*, **160(7)**: 1326–31.
The first large-scale study in the US of prevalence of eating disorders in a sample of black American young women. The study found no cases of AN in black women and a significantly lower number of cases of BN or BED in black women compared to white women. The authors caution, however, that the significantly later ages of onset of BN and BED in black women compared to white women may explain in part the lower prevalences of these disorders in this young adult sample.

*Sundgot-Borgen J and Torstveit MK (2004) Prevalence of eating disorders in elite athletes is higher than in the general population. *Clin J Sport Med*, **14(1)**: 25–32.

*Tolgyes T and Nemessury J (2004) Epidemiological studies on adverse dieting behaviours and eating disorders among young people in Hungary. *Soc Psychiatry Psychiatr Epidemiol*, **39(8)**: 647–54.

*von Ranson KM, McGue M and Iacono WG (2003) Disordered eating and substance use in an epidemiological sample: II. Associations within families. *Psychol Addict Behav*, **17(3)**: 193–201.

Wilfley DE, Schwartz MB, Spurrell EB and Fairburn CG (2000) Using the eating disorder examination to identify the specific psychopathology of binge eating disorder. *Int J Eat Disord*, **27(3)**: 259–69.

5

Body image

Leslie J Heinberg and J Kevin Thompson

Abstract

Objectives of review. The explosive growth in research in the area of body image has produced a wealth of work relevant to understanding eating disorders. This review will summarize the body image literature from 2003–2004 that specifically relates to eating disorders, eating behavior and dieting.

Summary of recent findings. Recent experimental, correlational and prospective studies not only indicate the predictive utility of body image measures in explaining eating disturbances, but also offer insights into the potential risk factors that illuminate the onset and perpetuation of body image problems. New assessment strategies have also emerged in the last two years and researchers are beginning to document the body image changes subsequent to an eating disorders treatment program.

Future directions. Future work needs to further evaluate the specific effects of body image treatment paradigms targeted toward eating disturbances, along with a renewed focus on whether the current definitional schemes for body image disturbance are optimal.

Introduction

Providing a summary of the last two years of body image research is a far greater challenge than it would have been as recently as five years ago. Cited references number 824 when using body image as the key word for a Medline search and limiting the dates to 2003 and 2004. By contrast, five years ago (1998–1999) there were 662 articles. A decade ago (1993–1994) there were 546 body image citations. This 150% increase in the literature attests to the exploding interest in body image as an important domain of research. Such growth and interest are particularly evident in the emergence of a new scholarly journal, *Body Image: An International Journal of Research*, devoted exclusively to the field.

This review will limit itself to selected articles that are most relevant to eating disorders, dieting, and eating behavior. However, it should be noted that there is growing interest in examining body image outside of the realm of eating behaviors and disorders in such diverse fields as medical populations, sexuality, anthropology and neurosciences (Pruzinsky and Cash 2002). Our literature review is broadly organized into the following sections: descriptive studies, etiology, assessment, prevention and treatment, and the predictive utility of body image.

Literature review

Descriptive studies

Studies that investigate the prevalence of body dissatisfaction (BD) or demographic differences in degree of BD continue to be a large focus of the literature. Of particular interest was the publication of a cross-sectional study examining body image from 1983 to 2001 (Cash *et al.* 2004b). Significant changes in the body image of college-aged men and women occurred over the 19-year period. Non-Black (predominantly White) women evidenced a worsening body image from the 1980s to mid-1990s. Conversely, Black women generally did not evince these changes. More recent non-Black and Black cohorts, however, reported a more favorable body image in spite of the population becoming heavier over time (Cash *et al.* 2004b). In contrast to Cash's findings based on the *Psychology Today* survey (Pruzinsky and Cash 2002), men's body image was remarkably stable over time. Striegel-Moore *et al.* (2004) prospectively evaluated body image changes in several eating disorder groups and controls at several time points: two years and then one year prior to the onset of the disorder, at the time of onset, and again, one year and then two years after onset of the eating disorder. Among a host of findings, they noted that the bulimia nervosa (BN) group had the highest weight dissatisfaction at all time points and the binge-eating disorder (BED) participants had higher dissatisfaction than the non-eating disordered controls.

A number of studies have continued to evaluate racial/ethnic differences (Perez and Joiner 2003; Freedman *et al.* 2004) or lack thereof (Shaw *et al.* 2004) in BD. In general, studies demonstrate differences in body image ideals and severity of BD, with ethnicities that endorse a broader range of acceptable body types also endorsing greater body size satisfaction. Ethnicity should continue to be a variable of interest and specific assessment of ethnicity rather than the use of gross categories should be included in future studies (Tsai *et al*. 2003; Yates *et al*. 2004).

There has been burgeoning interest in the role of sexual orientation and BD. For instance, studies have evaluated differences in body satisfaction and eating disturbance among homosexual and heterosexual men and women (Morrison *et al*. 2004) and boys and girls (Austin *et al*. 2004), the 'muscular ideal' endorsed by gay men (Yelland and Tiggemann 2003), and the influence of media consumption on straight and gay males' body image (Duggan and McCreary 2004). This study found that consumption of muscle and fitness magazines was positively related to body dissatisfaction in both gay and straight males, but pornography exposure was only related to physique anxiety in gay men.

Etiology

The majority of work in the field of body image over the past two years can be broadly defined as etiological in nature. We have previously organized theoretical explanations into four categories: (1) socialization by culture; (2) personality characteristics; (3) interpersonal experiences; and (4) activating events and situations (e.g. Thompson *et al*. 2005). The literature of the past two years will be addressed in order of these four organizing principles, after first reviewing a seminal study in the area of genetic influence.

Genetics

Genetic research is one of the most important and promising areas in the etiology of eating disorders. However, such research typically does not include examination of body image issues. Reichborn-Kjennerud *et al*. (2004) take a large step in filling this gap by exploring the heritability of 'undue influence of weight on self-evaluation' (an operationalization of body image that adheres closely to the DSM definition) in a sample of 8045 same-sex and opposite-sex Norwegian twins, aged 18–31. They found that shared environmental factors accounted for 31% of the variance in such body disturbance; non-shared or common environmental factors explained 69% of the variance. Although the authors could not address the nature of the shared environmental influences, they recommended that future work explore this issue, along with the possible interaction of environmental factors and genetic factors. In an accompanying commentary to the article, Schmidt (2004) noted the importance of focusing attention on the common factors, which might include media, peer, and parental influences (*see* also Thompson *et al*. 1999; van den Berg *et al*. 2002).

Socialization by culture

Body image researchers continue to focus on how sociocultural influences and the media affect BD in girls and women (Harrison 2003; Tiggemann and Slater 2003; Joshi et al. 2004). A positive change in the research direction is the recent work examining these influences in adolescent boys and in minority populations. Humphreys and Paxton (2004) showed that boys (mean age 15.6 years) with high internalization (e.g. endorsement) of the muscular, athletic ideal had more negative responses on body image and mood after exposure to idealized male images compared to adolescent boys low on internalization. Taveras and colleagues (2004) demonstrated that physical activity levels were higher by 1.2 hours per week in boys (and 0.7 hours for girls) for every 1 (out of 5) category increase in wanting to look like figures in the media. In a large ($n=4746$) population-based study, Utter et al. (2003) showed that, like girls, middle and high-school-aged boys reported frequent reading of magazine articles about dieting and weight loss and that frequent readers were more likely to be overweight, non-White, and lower SES. For both genders, frequent exposure to magazine articles was associated with greater weight loss behaviors and elevated psychosocial distress, findings maintained after controlling for differences in body satisfaction, self-esteem and depression. Finally, Hargreaves and Tiggemann (2003) found that exposing boys with moderate levels of appearance investment to commercials of women who epitomize the thin ideal led to boys rating appearance as a more important attribute when choosing a girl-friend/partner.

Schooler and colleagues (2004) found that viewing mainstream television predicted *poorer* body image for White women, but was unrelated to body image in Black women. Conversely, viewing Black-oriented media was unrelated to body image in White women, but predicted *healthier* body image in Black women.

Personality characteristics

Although the vast majority of individuals are exposed to the thin ideal and cultural expectations of femininity, researchers have begun to examine dispositional variables that may render persons at greater risk for sociocultural influences. Internalization of the thin ideal has received a significant amount of scholarly attention in the last two years (e.g. Hermes and Keel 2003; Low et al. 2003). Research continued to demonstrate the mediational role of internalization in the relationship between BMI and BD (Shroff and Thompson 2004), between awareness of thin ideals and BD (Sands and Wardle 2003), and between perceived pressure to be thin and BD (Blowers et al. 2003). In a path analytic study of middle school-aged girls evaluating the Tripartite Influence Model (peers, parents, media; *see* Thompson et al. 1999), internalization fully mediated the relationship between parental influence and BD and partially mediated both the relationship between peer influence and media influence on BD (Keery et al. 2004b). In contrast, in an experimental study in which a thin confederate complained how fat she was and discussed her desire to diet, internalization of the thin ideal did not moderate or mediate the relationship between exposure to the experimental condition and increased BD (Stice *et al.* 2003).

Tiggemann and Slater (2003) examined the influence of social comparison processing on BD after women viewed a videotape with music videos that promoted the thin ideal. Viewing music videos that feature thin, attractive women led to increased BD and social comparison but this effect was mediated by baseline levels of comparison processing. Comparison processing was determined by summing the degree to which individuals thought about their appearance while watching videos and the degree to which they compared themselves to the women in the videos. Finally, in a study examining both social comparison and internalization of the thin ideal, body-focused anxiety of adult women was investigated following exposure to a thin model, average-sized model, or a model absent condition (Dittmar and Howard 2004). Both social comparison tendency and internalization moderated media effects on body-focused anxiety. However, internalization was shown to be a more proximal and specific predictor than social comparison. High internalization undermined the positive effect of exposure to an average-size model when it occurred in combination with habitual social comparison (Dittmar and Howard 2004).

Interpersonal experiences

A number of theories of body image disturbance have examined the effect of close relationships on the development and persistence of body image problems. Teasing, family attitudes and peer and romantic relationships have all been examined as meaningful explanations of BD (Thompson *et al.* 2005). The relationship between BD and appearance-related teasing continues to receive support in the literature (Milkewicz *et al.* 2003). In an adolescent sample, Eisenberg and colleagues (2003) found that teasing about body weight from two sources was associated with a higher prevalence of emotional problems than either no teasing or teasing from a single source. A history of hurtful racial teasing was recently found to be associated with eating and body image disturbance, whereas acculturation was not (Sahi Iyer and Haslam 2003).

There has been increased interest in familial influences on body image in both children and adults (e.g. Ericksen *et al.* 2003; Palladino Green and Pritchard 2003). A couple of recent studies have also examined the influence of romantic partners on BD. After controlling for BMI, both familial and spousal body-focused commentary predicted BD (Pole *et al.* 2004). Markey and colleagues (2004) found that wives overestimate their husbands' dissatisfaction with the wives' bodies and that husbands' satisfaction with their wives' bodies was better predicted by wives' dissatisfaction than BMI. Cash and colleagues (2004d) found that a more secure attachment was significantly related to a greater body satisfaction and less dysfunctional investment in appearance for both the male and the female involved in a romantic relationship.

Activating events/situations

A number of life events and situations, such as pubertal timing and BMI, have been proposed as activating for BD. These activating variables received significant attention by researchers in the context of other variables in the last two years. For example, studies found that more developed girls had greater internalization of the thin ideal (Hermes and Keel 2003) and that, for boys, the main predictor of body change strategies was puberty (Ricciardelli *et al.* 2003).

Integrative studies

In a one-year longitudinal study of body image among adolescent boys and girls, internalization of a muscular ideal predicted the development of BD in boys (Carlson Jones 2004). However, the development of BD in girls was predicted by BMI, appearance conversations with friends, and social comparison tendencies (Carlson Jones 2004). McCabe and Ricciardelli (2003) evaluated the role of parents, peers and the media on body image among adolescents. For boys, sociocultural influences and feedback from one's best friend predicted body change strategies. For girls, sociocultural influences and feedback from one's best friend and mother predicted body change strategies. Keery *et al.* (2004b), using structural equation modeling, found that peer, parental and media influences had both direct and indirect effects (via internalization and appearance comparision) on BD and eating disturbance. Studies that integrate one or more theoretical explanations should be encouraged so that the differential effect of various explanations on body image may be better determined.

Assessment

The assessment of body image is often essential to the diagnosis and selection of treatment for eating disorders because a disturbance in body image is a required criterion for the diagnosis of anorexia nervosa (AN) and BN. Cash *et al.* (2004c) developed the Body Image Disturbance Questionnaire, a measure which goes beyond the typical measure of 'dissatisfaction' by providing information on the degree to which unhappiness with appearance has an impact upon psychological and social functioning. The measure converges well with measures of eating disturbance, self-esteem, and depression. It also predicts variance associated with psychosocial functioning beyond that accounted for by BD. Cash *et al.* (2004a) also developed an extension of the Appearance Schemas Inventory, which is now a 20-item scale with two subscales (self-evaluative salience and motivational salience) and excellent psychometric characteristics for both males and females. Thompson *et al.* (2003) developed the Body Image Guilt and Shame Scale. Both indices of body image were associated with physique anxiety, body image concern, and body image importance. Shafran *et al.* (2004) developed the Body Checking and Avoidance Questionnaire, which provides an index of two of the key behavioral indicators of body image disturbance. They found that eating-disordered patients scored higher on the scale than controls, and concluded that body checking and avoidance were direct expressions of the 'over-evaluation of shape and weight' (p. 93).

Other important innovations in body image assessment include the continuation of work by Gardner in the detection of sensory and nonsensory components of body image (Gardner and Boice 2004) and a recent focus on measurement issues involved in the assessment of body image in males (e.g. Cafri and Thompson 2004a,b). (For a further review of the new and formative work in the body image assessment area, *see* Thompson *et al*. 2005.)

Measures of putative risk factors for body image and eating disturbances also appeared in the last two years. The third version of the Sociocultural Attitudes Towards Appearance Questionnaire (SATAQ-3; Thompson *et al*. 2004) included three subscales reflecting various dimensions of a media influence: information, pressures, and internalization. Calogero *et al*. (2004) evaluated the measure in a large sample of individuals with eating disorders, finding that it had excellent reliability and validity. Keery *et al*. (2004a) developed a measure of internalization of media ideals specific for adolescents (Sociocultural Internalization of Appearance Questionnaire: Adolescents). Psychometric characteristics were found to be excellent in samples from the US, Australia, and India. Additionally, in all three countries levels of internalization were associated significantly with degree of eating disturbance. Keery *et al*. (2004b) factorially evaluated a variety of measures of peer, parental, and media influence in their test of the Tripartite Influence Model of body image and eating disturbance. This study improved upon previous work by providing an assessment measure that consisted of multiple aspects of peer, parental, and media influence. Their findings supported the Tripartite model, in that these influences had both direct and indirect effects (through social comparison and internalization) on body dissatisfaction and eating disturbances.

Prevention and treatment

A few studies appeared in the area of prevention and/or treatment of body image and eating problems. McVey and colleagues (2004) conducted a six-session school-based intervention in middle-school-aged girls to improve body image, self-esteem and eating behaviors. At post-intervention, body image, self-esteem and dieting attitudes were reduced. However, at six and 12 months, the intervention group did not differ from controls on body image and self-esteem, although reductions in disturbed eating attitudes and behaviors were maintained. Wade *et al*. (2003) compared a school-based media literacy program to a self-esteem enhancement group and a control group, finding that the media literacy had improved scores on weight concern versus the control group at post-intervention. However, there were no differential group effects on shape concern, dietary restriction, or body dissatisfaction.

Matusek *et al*. (2004) compared a dissonance induction and a health eating/exercise psychoeducational intervention; equivalent improvements for both groups were found for drive for thinness, thin-ideal internalization and eating behaviors. In an innovative Internet-based study, a professionally moderated Internet chat-room reduced eating pathology and self-esteem among college-aged women at risk for developing eating disorders (Zabinski *et al.* 2004).

A model to explain unhealthy weight-control behaviors in adolescents was developed and tested by Neumark-Sztainer and colleagues (2003) with specific recommendations for prevention programs in the school and community. Their findings suggest that prevention efforts need to focus on improving body image and decreasing weight concerns and changing weight-specific social norms within the peer and family environments. It is hoped that these theoretically based recommendations will result in better future prevention programs.

Regarding treatment, cognitive-behavioral group treatment for BN resulted in reductions in BD (Peterson *et al.* 2004) and cognitive-behavioral treatment with an exposure component versus a cognitive restructuring component equally improved body image among patients with BED (Hilbert and Tuchen-Caffier 2004).

Predictive utility of body image

The construct of body image continues to demonstrate utility in predicting the development, maintenance and severity of a wide variety of eating behaviors and disorders, and health behaviors.

Eating behaviors

Body image dissatisfaction has been shown to relate to chronic dieting (Gingras *et al.* 2004), higher dietary restraint in nine-year-old girls (Krahnstoever Davison *et al.* 2003), dieting behavior in adolescents (Børresen and Rosenvinge 2003), and intention to use weight loss products in spite of knowledge of their harmful effects (Whisenhunt *et al.* 2003).

Eating disorders

The importance of BD as a diagnostic criterion for AN (Kovacs and Palmer 2004) and BN (Perez and Joiner 2003) continued to receive support. Although long investigated in AN and BN, the role of body image in BED has recently garnered greater interest. For example, Masheb and Grilo (2003) found that self-evaluation unduly influenced by body shape was a greater indicator of BED than BD or self-evaluation unduly influenced by weight.

Health behaviors

The importance of body image in predicting health behaviors or engagement in risky health behaviors has received increasing attention. BD did not predict regular exercise in older adults (age 50–98; Schuler *et al.* 2004) but wanting to look like media figures did predict adolescent boys' and girls' physical activity (Taveras *et al.* 2004).

In a four-year prospective study of female adolescents aged 12–15 years at baseline, girls who valued thinness most strongly or somewhat strongly were more likely to become established smokers than girls who valued it least strongly (Honjo and Siegel 2003). These results were independent of age, race/ethnicity, and baseline smoking status. Similarly, Stice and Shaw (2003) showed that elevated eating pathology and BD predicted onset of smoking, but that negative affectivity did not. A recent review concluded that a positive relationship exists between smoking and dieting behaviors, disordered eating symptoms and weight concerns in adolescent girls but not boys (Potter *et al.* 2004).

Clinical implications

Research over the past two years supports a wide range of studies conducted over the past two decades indicating that it is critical to assess and evaluate body image disturbance for individuals with eating disorders. The studies reviewed herein indicate that body image remains closely connected to eating disturbances and many of the factors receiving support as possible risks for body image disturbances are also potentially associated with the onset or maintenance of eating disturbances (e.g. internalization of media images and messages). Studies on etiology and risk factors continue to support the integration of strategies targeting common environmental factors (media, peer, parental) into extant prevention programs. Prevention studies have benefited tremendously by an inclusion of strategies to reduce not only body image disturbances, but also other factors (such as internalization) thought to perpetuate negative body image.

The development of some new measures of assessment over the past two years, in particular the Body Image Disturbance Questionnaire, Body Checking and Avoidance Scale, and Body Image Guilt and Shame Scale, provides some new strategies that might be integrated into the assessment of eating disorders. These new scales, designed specifically to get at the extreme subjective, cognitive, and behavioral aspects of appearance (often found in individuals with eating disorders), might provide critical information for treatment prescription.

Future directions

Although research is proceeding at a vigorous pace in the areas of etiology and assessment, little progress has actually been made in the specific area of treatment of body image disturbances in individuals with eating disorders. As we noted 10 years ago (Thompson *et al.* 1996), eating disorder treatment manuals and empirically driven intervention strategies often fail to fully target the body image component; the situation has changed little in the time since we conducted that review. In a series of studies with his CBT program for body image, Cash and colleagues (for a review, *see* Cash and Hrabosky 2004) have found that such a treatment improves not only body image, but also eating disturbance. In a recent study, Nye and Cash (2004) found that individuals with a diagnosed eating disorder improved on measures of body image disturbance after receiving the body image CBT treatment.

Although work in the area of body image in men and the 'muscular ideal' has garnered recent attention (Cafri and Thompson 2004a,b; Cafri *et al*. 2005), relatively little work has evaluated the specific connection between body image issues for men and eating disturbances. Men who have a 'drive for muscularity' may exhibit eating patterns that are quite different from those often seen in men who restrict and/or purge to lose weight. Extreme carbohydrate depletion, supplement use, and steroid use are examples of behaviors that might be associated with body image disturbance, body dysmorphic disorder, or, in some cases, an eating disorder (although it might only meet criteria for the diagnosis of EDNOS). Much more work on the etiology, assessment, and treatment of body image issues and eating disturbances with men needs to be undertaken.

Finally, theoretical and empirical work needs to focus on operationalization of the body image construct with regard to its definition in the context of eating disorders. We have previously noted that the construct of 'body image' can actually be operationalized in many ways, with some definitions and terms reflecting the same underlying construct, and others reflecting unique aspects of appearance disturbance (Thompson *et al*. 1999; Thompson 2004). The operationalization of body image canonized in the DSM for AN and BN compounds this problem with its use of phrases such as 'self-evaluation is unduly influenced by body shape and weight' (BN) and 'undue influence of bodyweight or shape on self-evaluation' (AN). As eloquently put by Schmidt (2004), 'Self-evaluation is a rather complex concept and I wonder how well people understand this question without any further explanation or probes' (p. 133). Schmidt was referring directly to the Reichborn-Kjennerud *et al*. (2004) study, wherein participants were asked specifically, 'is it important for your self-evaluation that you keep a certain weight?' (p. 125); however, the question could also be asked of professionals and researchers in the field of body image and eating disorders. Clearly, one direction for the future is the evaluation of how we operationalize body image in our measures, and whether we need to reconsider our definition of the body image disturbance criterion for AN and BN.

Corresponding author: Leslie J Heinberg, Associate Professor, Department of Epidemiology and Biostatistics, Case Western Reserve University, 10900 Euclid Avenue/WG-72, Cleveland, OH 44106, USA. Email: leslie.heinberg@case.edu

References

References included from the targeted review years are preceded by one asterisk. References preceded by three asterisks are of particular significance. The significance is explained by a short commentary following the complete reference.

*Austin SB, Ziyadeh N, Kahn JA, Camargo CA, Coditz GA and Field AE (2004) Sexual orientation, weight concerns, and eating-disordered behaviors in adolescent girls and boys. *Journal of the American Academy of Child and Adolescent Psychiatry*, **43(9)**: 1115–23.

*Blowers LC, Loxton NJ, Grady-Flesser M, Occhipinti S and Dawe S (2003) The relationship between sociocultural pressure to be thin and body dissatisfaction in preadolescent girls. *Eating Behaviors*, **4(3)**: 229–44.

*Børresen R and Rosenvinge JH (2003) Body dissatisfaction and dieting in 4,952 Norwegian children aged 11–15 years: Less evidence for gender and age differences. *Eating and Weight Disorders*, **8**: 238–41.

*Cafri G and Thompson JK (2004a) Measuring male body image: A review of the current methodology. *Psychology of Men & Masculinity*, **5**: 18–29.

*Cafri G and Thompson JK (2004b) Evaluating the convergence of muscle appearance attitude measures. *Assessment*, **11**: 224–9.

***Cafri G, Thompson JK, Ricciardelli L, McCabe M, Smolak L and Yesalis C (2005) Pursuit of the muscular ideal: Physical and psychological consequences and putative risk factors. *Clinical Psychology Review*, **25**: 215–39.

This is a comprehensive review of the physical issues involved in the pursuit of the muscular ideal (e.g. steroid use, extreme carbohydrate depletion diets), along with the psychological consequences (e.g. depression) that flow from use, with a special focus on a model of putative risk factors, including family, peer, and media influences.

*Calogero RM, Davis WN and Thompson JK (2004) The Sociocultural Attitudes Towards Appearance Questionnaire (SATAQ-3): Reliability and normative comparisons of eating disordered patients. *Body Image: An International Journal of Research*, **1**: 193–8.

*Carlson Jones D (2004) Body image among adolescent girls and boys: A longitudinal study. *Developmental Psychology*, **40(5)**: 823–35.

*Cash TF and Hrabosky J (2004) Treatment of body image disturbance. In: JK Thompson (ed), *Handbook of Eating Disorders and Obesity*. John Wiley & Sons, New York, pp 515–41.

*Cash TF, Melnyk SE and Hrabosky JI (2004a) The assessment of body image investment: An extensive revision of the Appearance Schemas Inventory. *International Journal of Eating Disorders*, **35**: 305–16.

***Cash TF, Morrow JA, Hrabosky JI and Perry AA (2004b) How has body image changed? A cross-sectional investigation of college women and men from 1983 to 2001. *Journal of Consulting and Clinical Psychology*, **72(6)**: 1081–9.

This cross-sectional study examined changes in body image in 3127 college-aged men and women using standardized assessment across 22 studies over a 19-year period conducted at the same university. Two reliable patterns emerged: a worsening of body image in women from the 1980s until the mid-1990s followed by improvements in body image and a stability of men's body image over time.

*Cash TF, Phillips KA, Santos MT and Hrabosky JI (2004c) Measuring 'negative body image': Validation of the Body Image Disturbance Questionnaire in a nonclinical population. *Body Image: An International Journal of Research*, **1(4)**: 363–72.

*Cash TF, Thériault J and Milkewicz Annis N (2004d) Body image in an interpersonal context: Adult attachment, fear of intimacy, and social anxiety. *Journal of Social and Clinical Psychology*, **23(1)**: 89–103.

*Dittmar H and Howard S (2004) Thin-ideal internalization and social comparison tendency as moderators of media models' impact on women's body-focused anxiety. *Journal of Social and Clinical Psychology*, **23(6)**: 768–91.

*Duggan SJ and McCreary DR (2004) Body image, eating disorders, and the drive for muscularity in gay and heterosexual men: The influence of media images. *Journal of Homosexuality*, **47(3–4)**: 45–58.

*Eisenberg ME, Neumark-Sztainer D and Story M (2003) Associations of weight-based teasing and emotional well-being among adolescents. *Archives of Pediatric Adolescent Medicine*, **157(8)**: 733–8.

*Ericksen AJ, Markey CN and Tinsley BJ (2003) Familial influences on Mexican American and Euro-American preadolescents boys' and girls' body dissatisfaction. *Eating Behaviors*, **4(3)**: 245–55.

*Freedman RE, Carter MM, Sbrocco T and Gray JJ (2004) Ethnic differences in preference for female weight and waist-to-hip ratio: A comparison of African-American and White American college and community samples. *Eating Behaviors*, **5(3)**: 191–8.

*Gardner RM and Boice R (2004) A computer program for measuring body size distortion and body dissatisfaction. *Behavior Research Methods, Instruments, & Computers*, **36**: 89–95.

*Gingras J, Fitzpatrick J and McCargar L (2004) Body image of chronic dieters: Lowered appearance evaluation and body satisfaction. *Journal of the American Dietetic Association*, **104(10)**: 1589–92.

*Hargreaves DA and Tiggemann M (2003) Female 'thin ideal' media images and boys' attitudes toward girls. *Sex Roles*, **49(9/10)**: 539–44.

*Harrison K (2003) Television viewers' ideal body proportions: The case of the curvaceously thin woman. *Sex Roles*, **48(5-6)**: 255–64.

*Hermes SF and Keel PK (2003) The influence of puberty and ethnicity on awareness and internalization of the thin ideal. *International Journal of Eating Disorders*, **33(4)**: 465–7.

*Hilbert A and Tuschen-Caffier B (2004) Body image interventions in cognitive-behavioral therapy of binge-eating disorder: A component analysis. *Behaviour Research and Therapy*, **42(11)**: 1325–39.

*Honjo K and Siegel M (2003) Perceived importance of being thin and smoking initiation among young girls. *Tobacco Control*, **12(3)**: 289–95.

*Humphreys P and Paxton SJ (2004) Impact of exposure to idealized male images on adolescent boys' body image. *Body Image*, **1(3)**: 253–66.

*Joshi R, Herman CP and Polity J (2004) Self-enhancing effects of exposure to thin-body images. *International Journal of Eating Disorders*, **35**: 333–41.

*Keery H, Shroff H, Thompson JK, Wertheim E and Smolak L (2004a) The Sociocultural Internalization of Appearance Questionnaire – Adolescents (SIAQ-A): Psychometric and normative data for three countries. *Eating and Weight Disorders: Studies on Anorexia, Bulimia and Obesity*, **9**: 56–61.

***Keery H, van den Berg P and Thompson JK (2004b) An evaluation of the Tripartite Influence Model of body dissatisfaction and eating disturbance with adolescent girls. *Body Image*, **1(3)**: 237–51.

This study evaluated the role of three formative influences (media, peers, parents) in the formation of body dissatisfaction and eating disturbance in young adolescent females. Using structural equation modeling, the results indicated that the composite score of the influences led to body dissatisfaction and eating disturbance, and the effect was partially mediated by internalization of societal norms for appearance and appearance comparison tendencies.

Kovacs D and Palmer RL (2004) The associations between laxative abuse and other symptoms among adults with anorexia nervosa. *International Journal of Eating Disorders*, **36(2)**: 224–8.

*Krahnstoever Davison K, Markey CN and Birch LL (2003) A longitudinal examination of patterns in girls' weight concerns and body dissatisfaction from ages 5 to 9 years. *International Journal of Eating Disorders*, **33(3)**: 320–32.

*Low KG, Charanasomboon S, Brown C *et al*. (2003) Internalization of the thin ideal, weight and body image concerns. *Social Behavior and Personality*, **31(1)**: 81–90.

*Markey CN, Markey PM and Birch LL (2004) Understanding women's body satisfaction: The role of husbands. *Sex Roles*, **51(3–4)**: 209–16.

*Masheb RM and Grilo CM (2003) The nature of body image disturbance in patients with binge eating disorder. *International Journal of Eating Disorders*, **33(3)**: 333–41.

*Matusek JA, Wendt SJ and Wiseman CV (2004) Dissonance thin–ideal and didactic healthy behavior eating disorder prevention programs: Results from a controlled trial. *International Journal of Eating Disorders*, **36**: 376–88.

***McCabe MP and Ricciardelli LA (2003) Sociocultural influences on body image body changes among adolescent boys and girls. *Journal of Social Psychology*, **143(1)**: 5–26.
The authors evaluated the relative importance of parents, peers and the media in body image and body-change strategies among 622 adolescent boys and 644 adolescent girls. For boys, sociocultural influences and feedback from one's best friend predicted body change strategies. For girls, sociocultural influences and feedback from one's best friend and mother predicted body change strategies.

*McVey GL, Davis R, Tweed S and Shaw BF (2004) Evaluation of a school-based program designed to improve body image satisfaction, global self-esteem, and eating attitudes and behaviors: A replication study. *International Journal of Eating Disorders*, **36**: 1–11.

*Milkewicz Annis N, Cash TF and Hrabosky JI (2004) Body image and psychosocial differences among stable average weight, currently overweight, and formerly overweight women: The role of stigmatizing experiences. *Body Image*, **1(2)**: 155–67.

*Morrison MA, Morrison TG and Sager C (2004) Does body dissatisfaction differ between gay men and lesbian women and heterosexual men and women? A meta-analytic review. *Body Image*, **1(2)**: 127–38.

*Morrison TG, Kalin R and Morrison MA (2004) Body-image evaluation and body-image investment among adolescents: A test of sociocultural and social comparison theories. *Adolescence*, **39(155)**: 571–91.

*Neumark-Sztainer D, Wall MM, Story M and Perry CL (2003) Correlates of unhealthy weight-control behaviors among adolescents: Implications for prevention programs. *Health Psychology*, **22(1)**: 88–98.

*Neumark-Sztainer D, Goeden C, Story M and Wall M (2004) Associations between body satisfaction and physical activity in adolescents: Implications for programs aimed at preventing a broad spectrum of weight-related disorders. *Eating Disorders*, **12**: 125–37.

Nye S and Cash TF (2004) Outcomes of manualized cognitive-behavioral body image therapy with eating disordered women treated in a private clinical practice. Unpublished manuscript.

*Palladino Green S and Pritchard ME (2003) Predictors of body image dissatisfaction in adult men and women. *Social Behavior and Personality*, **31(3)**: 215–22.

*Perez M and Joiner TE (2003) Body image dissatisfaction and disordered eating in black and white women. *International Journal of Eating Disorders*, **33**: 342–50.

*Peterson CB, Wimmer S, Ackard DM *et al*. (2004) Changes in body image during cognitive-behavioral treatment in women with bulimia nervosa. *Body Image*, **1(2)**: 139–53.

*Pole M, Crowther JH and Schell J (2004) Body dissatisfaction in married women: The role of spousal influence and marital communication patterns. *Body Image*, **1(3)**: 267–78.

*Potter BK, Pederson LL, Chan SS, Aubut JA and Koval JJ (2004) Does a relationship exist between body weight, concerns about weight, and smoking among adolescents? An integration of the literature with an emphasis on gender. *Nicotine and Tobacco Research*, **6(3)**: 397–425.

Pruzinsky T and Cash TF (2002) Understanding body images: historical and contemporary perspectives. In: TF Cash and T Pruzinsky (eds), *Body Image: a handbook of theory, research and clinical practice*. Guilford Press, New York.

***Reichborn-Kjennerud T, Bulik CM, Kendler KS *et al*. (2004) Undue influence of weight on self-evaluation: A population-based twin study of gender differences. *International Journal of Eating Disorders*, **35**: 123–32.

One of the first studies to evaluate the shared versus nonshared environmental influences on the key DSM criterion related to body-image disturbance. A sample of over 8000 individuals was evaluated, with the results indicating that over two-thirds of the variance associated with body-image disturbance could be explained by common (nonshared) environmental factors.

*Ricciardelli LA, McCabe MP, Holt KE and Finemore J (2003) A biopsychosocial model for understanding body image and body change strategies among children. *Journal of Applied Developmental Psychology*, **24(4)**: 475–95.

*Sahi Iyer D and Haslam N (2003) Body image and eating disturbance among south Asian-American women: The role of racial teasing. *International Journal of Eating Disorders*, **34**: 142–7.

*Sands ER and Wardle J (2003) Internalization of ideal body shapes in 9–12-year-old girls. *International Journal of Eating Disorders*, **33**: 193–204.

Schmidt U (2004) Undue influence of weight on self-evaluation: A population-based twin study of gender differences. *International Journal of Eating Disorders*, **35**: 133–5.

Schooler D, Ward ML, Merriwether A and Caruthers A (2004) Who's that girl: Television's role in the body image development of young white and black women. *Psychology of Women Quarterly*, **28(1)**: 38–47.

Schuler PB, Broxon-Hutcherson A, Philipp SF *et al*. (2004) Body-shape perceptions in older adults and motivations for exercise. *Perceptual and Motor Skills*, **98(3)**: 1251–60.

*Shafran R, Fairburn CG, Robinson P and Lask B (2004) Body checking and its avoidance in eating disorders. *International Journal of Eating Disorders*, **35**: 93–101.

*Shaw H, Ramirez L, Trost A, Randall P and Stice E (2004) Body image and eating disturbances across ethnic groups: More similarities than differences. *Psychology of Addictive Behaviors*, **18(1)**: 12–18.

*Shroff H and Thompson JK (2004) Body image and eating disturbance in India: Media and interpersonal influences. *International Journal of Eating Disorders*, **35**: 198–203.

*Stice E and Shaw H (2003) Prospective relations of body image, eating and affective disturbances to smoking onset in adolescent girls: How Virginia slims. *Journal of Consulting and Clinical Psychology*, **71(1)**: 129–35.

*Stice E, Maxfield J and Wells T (2003) Adverse effects of social pressure to be thin on young women: An experimental investigation of the effects of 'fat talk'. *International Journal of Eating Disorders*, **34**: 108–17.

*Striegel-Moore RH, Franko DL, Thompson D, Barton B, Schreiber GB and Daniels SR (2004) Changes in weight and body image over time in women with eating disorders. *International Journal of Eating Disorders*, **36**: 315–27.

*Taveras EM, Rifas-Shiman SL, Field AE, Frazier AL, Colditz GA and Gillman MW (2004) The influence of wanting to look like media figures on adolescent physical activity. *Journal of Adolescent Health*, **35**: 41–50.

*Thompson JK (2004) The (mis)measurement of body image: ten strategies for improving assessment for research and clinical purposes. *Body Image: An International Journal of Research*, **1**: 7–14.

*Thompson JK, Heinberg LJ and Clarke AJ (1996) Treatment of body image disturbance in eating disorders. In: JK Thompson (ed), *Body Image, Eating Disorders and Obesity: an integrative guide for assessment and treatment*. American Psychological Association, Washington DC, pp 303–20.

*Thompson JK, Heinberg LJ, Altabe MN and Tantleff-Dunn S (1999) *Exacting Beauty: theory, assessment and treatment of body image disturbance*. American Psychological Association, Washington DC.

*Thompson JK, van den Berg P, Roehrig M, Guarda A and Heinberg LJ (2004) The Sociocultural Attitudes Towards Appearance Questionnaire-3 (SATAQ-3). *International Journal of Eating Disorders*, **35**: 293–304.

*Thompson JK, Roehrig M, Cafri G and Heinberg LJ (2005) Assessment of body image. In: JE Mitchell and CB Peterson (eds), *Assessment of Patients with Eating Disorders*. Guilford Press, New York.

*Thompson T, Dinnel DL and Dill NJ (2003) Development and validation of a Body Image Guilt and Shame Scale. *Personality and Individual Differences*, **34**: 59–75.

*Tiggemann M and Slater A (2003) Thin ideals in music television: A source of social comparison and body dissatisfaction. *International Journal of Eating Disorders*, **35**: 48–58.

*Tsai G, Curbow B and Heinberg LJ (2003) Sociocultural and developmental influences on body dissatisfaction and disordered eating attitudes and behaviors of Asian women. *Journal of Nervous and Mental Disease*, **191**: 309–18.

*Utter J, Neumark-Sztainer D, Wall M and Story M (2003) Reading magazine articles about dieting and associated weight control behaviors among adolescents. *Journal of Adolescent Health*, **32**: 78–82.

van den Berg P, Thompson JK, Brandon K and Coovert M (2002) The tripartite model of body image and eating disturbance: a covariance structure modeling investigation. *Journal of Psychosomatic Research*, **53**: 1007–20.

*Wade TD, Davidson and O'Dea JA (2003) A preliminary controlled evaluation of a school-based media literacy program and self-esteem program for reducing eating disorder risk factors. *International Journal of Eating Disorders*, **33**: 371–83.

*Whisenhunt BL, Williamson DA, Netemeyer RG and Andrews C (2003) Health risks, past usage, and intention to use weight loss products in normal weight women with high and low body dysphoria. *Eating and Weight Disorders*, **8**: 114–23.

*Yates A, Edman J and Aruguete M (2004) Ethnic differences in BMI and body/self-dissatisfaction among Whites, Asian subgroups, Pacific Islanders, and African-Americans. *Journal of Adolescent Health*, **34(4)**: 300–07.

*Yelland C and Tiggemann M (2003) Muscularity and the gay ideal: Body dissatisfaction and disordered eating in homosexual men. *Eating Behaviors*, **4(2)**: 107–16.

*Zabinski MF, Wilfley DE, Calfas KJ, Winzelberg AJ and Taylor CB (2004) An interactive psychoeducational intervention for women at risk of developing an eating disorder. *Journal of Consulting and Clinical Psychology*, **72(5)**: 914–19.

6

Personality and eating disorders

Drew Westen, Heather Thompson-Brenner and Joanne Peart

Abstract

Objectives of review. The objective of this chapter is to examine the current state of research on personality traits, personality disorders, and personality subtypes in eating disorders (EDs).

Summary of recent findings. Personality pathology, whether relatively mild or severe, is nearly ubiquitous in ED patients. Patients with EDs tend to have problems with negative affect, whether allied with perfectionism, anxious obsessionality, and overcontrol of impulses and emotions (often seen in restricting anorexia); or with emotional dysregulation, rejection sensitivity, and undercontrol of impulses and emotions (often seen in patients with bulimic symptoms, with or without anorexic features). Data using several methods have converged on three personality subtypes that appear to cut across different ED diagnoses, but have implications for understanding and treating patients with EDs.

Future directions. Although data are converging on several key constructs in the study of personality in EDs, different measures may be tapping different constructs or subconstructs, suggesting the need for research employing a range of measures of similar constructs in the same sample. Given the ubiquity of personality pathology in EDs and data suggesting that personality may moderate treatment response, it would seem prudent for all treatment research on EDs to assess personality carefully and to consider personality variables when constructing treatments for EDs.

Introduction

The earliest systematic clinical accounts of eating disorders (EDs) in the 1970s suggested a link between personality and EDs. Empirical developments in the study of EDs and of psychopathology more broadly (Krueger 2002; Kendler *et al.* 2003; Westen, Gabbard and Blagov in press) have recently borne out the importance of studying psychopathology in the context of personality. However, characterizing the precise nature of the link between personality and EDs poses a number of challenges.

Causal arrows linking eating and personality can run in multiple directions (*see* Bloks *et al.* 2004; Lilenfeld *et al.* in press; Stice *et al.* in press). Personality could predispose individuals to EDs; EDs could affect personality (e.g. patients with anorexia nervosa (AN) could become more obsessional while starving); or personality and eating pathology could mutually influence each other. Although the evidence is not definitive, and the causal arrows are surely multidirectional, personality variables do appear to represent diatheses for EDs. Recent prospective studies implicate neuroticism and its close cousin negative emotionality (Ghaderi and Scott 2000; Stice 2002; Cervera *et al.* 2003), obsessive–compulsive personality features (Lilenfeld *et al.* in press); impulsivity (Wonderlich *et al.* 2004), perfectionism (Bulik *et al.* 2003; Sherry *et al.* 2004), and poor interoceptive awareness (Lilenfeld *et al.* in press) as risk factors for EDs. Further research is necessary, however, to establish both the temporal relations and precise processes through which personality processes contribute to disordered eating (*see* Wonderlich *et al.* 2005a,b).

In this chapter we review three primary ways in which researchers have conceptualized and studied personality in EDs. We then discuss the clinical implications of recent research. We conclude by discussing future directions.

Literature review

Personality refers to enduring patterns of cognition, emotion, motivation, and behavior that are activated over time or circumstance. These patterns may express themselves in many situations (e.g. a tendency to feel inadequate) or may repeatedly express themselves only under certain very specific conditions (e.g. a tendency to choose troubled or inappropriate romantic partners). Researchers have conceptualized and studied personality in EDs in three ways, focusing on personality *traits*, *disorders*, and *subtypes*. We examine each in turn.

Personality traits

Traits are emotional, cognitive, and behavioral tendencies on which individuals vary (e.g. the tendency to experience negative emotions). Researchers studying personality traits in EDs tend either to focus on traits first observed clinically in ED patients or to compare different kinds of ED patients using trait dimensions assessed in omnibus personality inventories.

Three clinically observed traits have received substantial empirical attention. Two – perfectionism and obsessionality – were first identified in AN patients, and one – impulsivity – in bulimia nervosa (BN) patients. Studies have consistently reported significant comorbidity between EDs and obsessive–compulsive disorder (OCD) (e.g. Halmi *et al.* 2003). Obsessive–compulsive personality traits in childhood are highly predictive of subsequent ED development (Anderluh *et al.* 2003). Although the data are not yet conclusive as to the causal sequence linking obsessionality and EDs, a number of studies strongly suggest that obsessionality predates and is a significant risk factor for eating pathology (Anderluh *et al.* 2003). Compulsive and inhibited traits in ED patients also appear to be associated with distinct biological correlates, particularly in serotonergic functioning (Steiger *et al.* 2003; Bruce *et al.* 2004).

Whereas compulsivity has been most frequently identified in anorexia patients, impulsivity is more common in bulimia patients than either restricting AN patients (e.g. Vervaet *et al.* 2004) or normal comparison subjects (Kane *et al.* 2004). A widely studied distinction is between multi-impulsive and uni-impulsive bulimia (Lacey and Evans 1986). Multi-impulsive individuals with BN display several forms of impulsive behaviors (e.g. stealing, substance abuse) in addition to binge eating, whereas uni-impulsive patients only binge and purge. Empirically, multi-impulsive bulimic individuals tend to have significantly more psychopathology than uni-impulsive patients, particularly borderline personality disorder (BPD) and mood disorders (Fichter *et al.* 1994; Bell and Newns 2002). The uni/multi-impulsive distinction has been replicated cross-culturally: Matsunaga and colleagues (2000) found a multi-impulsive group in a sample of Japanese bulimia patients. Like their Western counterparts, this group also had a greater prevalence of BPD than uni-impulsive bulimics. Data on impulsivity appear to be particularly important in light of research linking impulsivity to early drop-out rates from psychotherapy (Agras *et al.* 2000).

Studies using omnibus trait measures have tended to produce a similar portrait of AN patients to that painted by studies of clinically observed traits: high in negative affectivity or neuroticism (anxious, fearful, and harm avoidant) and obsessionality (persistent). These results have begun to replicate cross-culturally, particularly for restricting AN (Nagata *et al.* 2003). BN patients, on the other hand, do not seem to fit any single profile. Like AN patients, they tend to be high in negative affectivity. However, some studies have shown bulimia patients to resemble AN patients in other respects, whereas others have found them to be more extraverted, impulsive, novelty seeking, and reward dependent (for similar cross-cultural data, *see* Nagata *et al.* 2003; Vervaet *et al.* 2004). Emerging research has begun to link both the compulsivity and perfectionism seen in AN patients and the impulsivity often seen in BN patients with serotonin dysregulation (e.g. Kaye *et al.* 2003).

Personality disorders

A second way in which researchers have examined personality in ED patients is by assessing personality disorders as defined by axis II of the *Diagnostic and*

Statistical Manual of Mental Disorders, 4th edition (DSM-IV). Whereas Cluster A (odd–eccentric) diagnoses are infrequent in ED samples, Cluster C (anxious–fearful) disorders are frequently observed in AN patients, and Cluster B (dramatic–erratic) in BN patients. Research suggests that Cluster C PDs are the most common among patients with all ED diagnoses, while Cluster B disorders are only present in those with bulimic symptomatology (Ilkjaer *et al.* 2004).

Borderline personality disorder is particularly common among binge-purging AN and BN patients (Skodol *et al.* 1993; Braun *et al.* 1994; Vitousek and Manke 1994). Conversely, EDs are very common in BPD samples. A recent prospective follow-up study of 290 BPD patients (Zanarini *et al.* 2004) found that, within six years of initial BPD diagnosis, 34% had met the criteria for a specific eating disorder and an additional 28% for eating disorder not otherwise specified (EDNOS). Among those whose BPD had remitted at six-year follow-up, rates of eating pathology declined from 55% to 26%. For nonremitting BPD patients, EDs were relatively stable (approximately 50%).

Personality subtypes

Research on axis II comorbidity in EDs tends to echo both the consistencies and inconsistencies in the literature using other personality constructs, such as traits (see Milos *et al.* 2003, 2004). Patients with AN, particularly restricting AN, tend to be avoidant (i.e. higher in negative affectivity and harm avoidance, and lower in extraversion) and obsessional (higher on rigidity, constraint, and compulsivity). Patients with BN are more likely to have borderline features (including negative affectivity, impulsivity, extraversion), although in some samples they are distinguished from other ED patients by their relative freedom from personality pathology. Complicating matters, binge-purging AN patients sometimes resemble AN patients and sometimes resemble BN patients, and most ED patients 'cross over' from AN to BN or vice versa at some point in their lives (Eddy *et al.* 2002), raising questions about how the two classes of ED could have differing personality profiles.

The combination of consistency and inconsistency in the literature has led to the hypothesis that patients with similar ED diagnoses may be heterogeneous vis-à-vis several distinct personality *styles,* that only imperfectly map onto DSM-IV ED diagnoses (Westen and Harden-Fischer 2001). Several research groups have attempted to cluster ED patients empirically based on personality data, and a convergence across methods has begun to emerge (Goldner *et al.* 1999; Westen and Harnden-Fischer 2001; Espelage *et al.* 2002; Thompson-Brenner and Westen 2005c; Wonderlich *et al.* 2005a). Although it is unclear to what extent patients classified using one instrument map onto those classified using a different measure, studies have generally identified three personality styles common among ED patients. The first is a *high functioning* style, sometimes allied with perfectionism and negative affectivity (Westen and Harnden-Fischer 2001; Wonderlich *et al.* 2005a). This style is most commonly seen in a subset of BN patients. The second is a *constricted, emotionally restrictive* style, most commonly observed in AN patients, with or without bulimic symptoms. Perfectionism and negative affect have also characterized this group in recent analyses (Wonderlich *et al.* 2005b). The third is an *impulsive* or *emotionally dysregulated* style, most often seen in patients with BN, with or without AN symptoms.

Across samples, the three subtypes differ in frequency of specific axis II symptoms in ways that make sense of the consistencies and inconsistencies in the literature. Compulsive/constricted patients, who are likely to have a diagnosis of restricting AN, tend to receive diagnoses of avoidant PD and obsessive compulsive personality disorder (OCPD). Impulsive/dysregulated patients, who are likely to have either BN or AN-BP, are most likely to have a diagnosis of BPD. High-functioning patients, who are most likely to have BN, are least likely to receive a PD diagnosis. These data make sense of the consistent findings of constricted personality traits in restricting anorexics, borderline and impulsive traits in a subset of patients with BN and AN-BP, and negative affectivity without a PD diagnosis in a subset of patients with both BN and anorexia nervosa-restricting type (AN-R).

Recent research has begun to flesh out the nature of these subtypes. In a sample of patients with BN symptoms patients treated in the community (Thompson-Brenner and Westen 2005a,b,c) showed high levels of constricted (31%) and dysregulated (27%) pathology, with the vast majority of patients (84%) readily classified by their treating clinicians into one of the three subtypes. Several studies have identified differences among the subtypes suggestive of a valid diagnostic distinction using Robins and Guze (1970) criteria, including differences in adaptive functioning, as reflected in Global Assessment of Functioning (GAF) scores and rates of hospitalization (Thompson-Brenner and Westen 2005a,c); variables relevant to etiology, such as childhood sexual abuse and family functioning (Eddy *et al.* 2004b; Thompson-Brenner and Westen 2005a,c); axis I and II comorbidity (Thompson-Brenner and Westen 2005a,c; Wonderlich *et al.* 2005a); adult sexual behavior (Eddy *et al.* 2004a); emotion regulation strategies (Harnden-Fischer *et al.* 2005; Wonderlich *et al.* 2005b); biology, including serotonin activity and neuro-psychological functioning (Bruce *et al.* 2004; Steiger *et al.* 2003, 2004); and treatment length and outcome (Thompson-Brenner and Westen 2005b,c). For example, in a naturalistic sample, constricted patients on average attained recovery approximately five months later than high-functioning patients, and dysregulated patients attained recovery approximately five months later than that (Thompson-Brenner and Westen 2005c). The percentage of patients who recovered (i.e. ceased bingeing and purging) during treatment was lower in the dysregulated group (43%), followed by the constricted (50%) and high-functioning groups (62%).

An alternative approach to subtyping has grouped ED patients into two clusters, described as 'dietary-alone' and 'dietary-negative affect', which show consistent differences in rates of associated personality pathology (Stice and Agras 1999; Grilo *et al.* 2001; Stice and Fairburn 2003). Compared with dietary-alone, the dietary-negative affect subtype shows higher rates of personality disorders; higher rates of mood, anxiety, and impulse control disorders; lower self-esteem; and increased social maladjustment.

Most recently, Grilo (2004) found that female adolescent psychiatric inpatients with features of EDs could be clustered into the same two groups.

The dietary-negative affective group (43%) was again characterized by higher levels of personality disturbance. As with personality pathology in EDs more generally, however, some of the elevations observed by Grilo appear somewhat inconsistent. For example, the dietary-negative affect group showed elevations in a set of scales reflecting anxious, avoidant, or internalizing pathology (e.g. inhibition, introversion, dolefulness) as well as other scales suggesting impulsive or externalizing pathology (e.g. oppositionality, borderline PD) (Grilo 2004). It may be that these apparent contradictions would be resolved by a three-cluster rather than a two-cluster solution, which distinguishes more disturbed patients with negative affectivity who are either constricted and overcontrolled from those who are impulsive and undercontrolled.

Summary of important findings

Personality pathology, whether relatively mild or severe, is nearly ubiquitous in EDs. Patients with EDs tend to have problems with negative affect, whether allied with perfectionism, anxious obsessionality, or the kinds of self-loathing, rejection sensitivity, and abandonment fears characteristic of patients with BPD. ED patients also tend to struggle with impulse and affect regulation. Some over-regulate their feelings, desires, and impulses; this is the case with many patients with the AN, restricting type. Others under-regulate, or have difficulty putting the brakes on their feelings, desires, and impulses; this appears to be the case with a substantial minority of patients with bulimic symptoms, whether diagnosed with BN, AN, binge-purging type or EDNOS. Data on personality subtypes suggest that we should not assume a one-to-one correspondence between symptoms and personality, and should correspondingly expect that the same disorder (e.g. BN) could be associated with both undercontrol and overcontrol, depending on sample characteristics (e.g. college student samples, where we might expect more high-functioning patients among those with BN than in an outpatient or hospital sample). To put it another way, the heterogeneity of personality with ED diagnoses (e.g. BN, or AN, binge-purge type) may be patterned, not random.

Clinical implications

Although we focus here primarily on treatment implications, an important implication for clinical assessment should be clear: clinicians treating ED patients should comprehensively assess patients' personality functioning as well as their eating (and other axis I) symptoms. The increasing body of literature linking personality to virtually all the disorders on axis I of DSM-IV suggests the importance of a comprehensive case formulation in treating ED and other patients.

Over the last decade, with the advent of the empirically supported therapies movement, research has focused on specific treatments for specific disorders, particularly cognitive–behavioral therapy (CBT) and interpersonal psychotherapy

(IPT) for BN. Data from randomized controlled trials (RCTs) for treatments for AN are more sparse (but beginning to emerge). Researchers have examined the moderating role of personality on treatment response for several years, at least for BN patients. The literature is by no means entirely consistent (*see* Bossert *et al.* 1992; Bulik *et al.* 1998; Grilo *et al.* 2003), likely reflecting a number of factors, including lack of power to detect differences, lack of data on personality, differences across studies in inclusion and exclusion criteria, and perhaps most importantly, the fact that virtually all RCTs have excluded certain patients with severe PDs either explicitly or *de facto* (e.g. excluding patients with substance abuse and suicidality, which eliminates most BPD patients; *see* Thompson-Brenner *et al.* 2003). Nevertheless, the outlines of a pattern emerge from the majority of studies. Several studies suggest that the presence of Cluster B (particularly borderline) pathology is associated with negative outcome (e.g. Johnson *et al.* 1990; Davis *et al.* 1992; Fahy and Russell 1993; Fairburn *et al.* 1993a; Rossiter *et al.* 1993; Wonderlich *et al.* 1994; Steiger and Stotland 1996). Related findings suggest that trait anger and impulsivity predict early drop-out from treatment (Fassino *et al.* 2003), and that negative emotionality, stress reactivity, and alienation predict low treatment-seeking behavior (Perkins *et al.* 2005). Other studies suggest that perfectionism, obsessive–compulsive PD, and asceticism also predict poor outcome in AN (e.g. Bizeul *et al.* 2001; Fassino *et al.* 2001; Rastam *et al.* 2003; Sutandar-Pinnock *et al.* 2003) (*see* Steinhausen 2002 for a review). It is of note that the two forms of severe personality disturbance identified in subtyping studies – constriction and impulsivity/dysregulation – both seem to be associated with poorer prognosis in RCTs. It is also of note that a trait associated with healthier forms of personality adaptation, 'self-directedness', predicts positive outcome (Fassino *et al.* 2003, 2004).

Research on personality has contributed to three new lines of research on treatment in ED patients. The first is the application of dialectical behavior therapy (DBT) to EDs. DBT is based on the rationale that emotional dysregulation is the core pathology in BPD, causing secondary disruptions in identity and interpersonal functioning (Linehan 1993; Linehan *et al.* 2001; McMain *et al.* 2001). DBT includes group and individual therapy, crisis intervention, and skills training. Abridged versions of DBT (fewer sessions per week, uni-modal treatment) have been tested with BN and binge-eating disorder (BED) (Safer *et al.* 2001; Telch *et al.* 2000, 2001). These reports suggest useful modifications of the DBT protocol for patients with eating symptoms, including expanded diary cards, nutritional education, and application of distress tolerance techniques to bodily focused judgments and impulses to binge (Wisniewski and Kelly 2003). In one study, DBT for BN produced substantial improvement, although recovery rates were not high relative to trials of CBT for BN (Safer *et al.* 2001). As several reviewers have suggested, research on DBT for BN and other EDs needs to identify the subgroups of patients who are most likely to benefit from DBT interventions, particularly given that many BN patients have more constricted forms of personality for which DBT may not be as useful (Kotler *et al.* 2003; Westen and Harnden-Fisher 2001). One case series has studied DBT with patients with severe, comorbid BN and BPD (Palmer *et al.* 2003). The therapy was effective in reducing days of inpatient hospitalization, self-harm, and ED symptoms, although three of five patients with BN continued to meet criteria for an ED post treatment. Nonetheless, the low drop-out rate and symptomatic improvement in this very severe sample suggest that elements of DBT may be useful for the treatment of dysregulated BN patients.

The second line of research in ED treatment relevant to personality is the development of enhanced, flexible, pan-disorder treatment manuals. The development of these manuals reflects the repeated observation that the relatively nonspecific diagnosis of EDNOS is the most prevalent ED in practice as well as the consistent observation of links between many forms of eating pathology and personality traits such as perfectionism, low self-esteem, difficulties with emotion regulation, and interpersonal problems (Fairburn *et al*. 2003). The basic formulation of BN reflected in the Fairburn *et al*. (1993b) CBT manual (CBT-93) is that overvaluation of shape and weight drives dietary restriction; dietary restriction leads to binge eating; and binge eating leads to compensatory behaviors that in turn produce additional vulnerability to binge eating. The new transdiagnostic treatment proposed by Fairburn and colleagues supplements this formulation, suggesting that several additional deficits may help maintain ED symptoms, including mood intolerance, interpersonal difficulties, low self-esteem, and clinical perfectionism (Fairburn *et al*. 2003, 2004). Although these deficits are not explicitly described as personality characteristics, they meet most definitions of personality (i.e. patterns of cognition, thought, and affect that persist across time or situation). The CBT-Enhanced (CBT-E) manual, which includes optional modules for each of these four deficits, is currently being tested with a transdiagnostic ED sample. Data collected to date on CBT-E with BN suggest that the treatment produces improvement and recovery in a greater percentage of cases (72%) than CBT-93 has in most prior BN samples (approximately 50%) (Fairburn 2004).

The third line of research has begun to use naturalistic data to study the influence of personality on treatments in the community (Thompson-Brenner and Westen 2005a,b,c). In a national sample of BN patients described by their treating clinician, personality subtype (dysregulated, constricted) showed systematic relations to the ways clinicians reported intervening with patients. The two most striking findings were a substantially increased use of intervention strategies associated with psychodynamic approaches among cognitive–behavioral (CBT) clinicians when working with dysregulated patients, and a shift toward more structured CBT interventions among psychodynamic clinicians when working with constricted patients. For CBT clinicians, the extent to which the patient showed evidence of dysregulation was correlated around $r=.50$ with their endorsement of statements such as the following: 'Helped the patient come to terms with her relationships with and feelings about significant others from the past (e.g. mother, father)'; 'Focused on similarities between the patient's relationships (and perceptions of relationships) repeated over time, settings, or people'; 'Addressed the patient's avoidance of important topics and shifts in mood'; 'Focused on the relationship between the therapist and patient'; and 'Focused on the influence of unconscious processes on behavior, emotions, beliefs'. For clinicians who reported a psychodynamic orientation, the extent to which the patient showed a constricted style correlated around $r=.30$ with the extent to which they reported that they 'taught the patient specific techniques for coping with her symptoms' and 'actively initiated the topics of discussion and other therapeutic activities'; and correlated $r=-.30$ with the item, 'Preferred that the patient, rather than the therapist, initiate the discussion of significant issues'. In addition, for clinicians of all theoretical orientations, patients' dysregulation was associated with use of adjunctive treatments, such as medication, group treatment, and hospitalizations. Multivariate analyses controlling for personality style found that use of CBT was associated with faster change in ED symptoms, while analyses controlling for personality style and treatment length found that psychodynamic therapy was associated with increased change in global functioning. Other recent naturalistic survey research finds that clinicians do not use structured treatment manuals because of their perceived inadequacy in addressing comorbidity (Haas and Clopton 2003), something that may perhaps change as research expands on CBT-E.

Future directions

These are clearly exciting times in the study of personality and EDs. What began with prescient clinical observations has become an increasingly sophisticated empirical literature on the relation between personality and eating pathology. In some ways, the study of personality in eating disorders, like the study of internalizing and externalizing personality spectra in axis I disorders (Krueger 2002), has taken us 'back to the future', to the idea that symptoms often need to be understood in their characterological context (Westen *et al.* in press). This does not mean returning to pre-empirical days of relying exclusively on clinical hunches about character structure or etiology. Rather, we are witnessing a period in which we may find substantial clinical and empirical utility in trying to bridge the chasm between decades-old clinical ideas about the way personality patterns may provide fertile ground for the development and maintenance of certain forms of psychopathology and contemporary research on the structure, behavioral genetics, and molecular genetics of personality and psychopathology.

The research described here suggests multiple directions for the future, of which we note two. First, although data are converging on several key constructs in the study of personality in EDs, we cannot assume that all measures purporting to assess the same construct are in fact doing so or doing so equally well. For example, impulsivity is a multidimensional construct, and measurement can focus on trait aspects associated with externalizing pathology, specific behaviors, or specific behaviors as indicators of latent traits (*see* Wonderlich *et al.* 2004). Similarly, although we have emphasized the convergence of different approaches to subtyping personality in EDs, the subtypes are not identical, and we cannot assume that self-report measures are assessing the same constructs as measures that require clinically experienced raters. There is good reason to believe that the assessment of personality pathology can be complicated by patients' lack of insight and by their lack of expertise in assessing constructs such as regulation of emotion, identification and tolerance of affect, and subtle aspects of interpersonal functioning (e.g. the extent to which the person can form rich and nuanced representations of the self and others) (*see* Westen 1997). Perhaps the best strategy at this point would be to collect data using multiple instruments and observers on the range of personality constructs studied in EDs to assess convergence and to conduct analyses across instruments to identify common dimensions as in recent research on the major self-report personality trait instruments (Markon *et al*. 2005).

Second, as a field, we are only beginning to grapple with personality as a variable of importance in the treatment of EDs. Preliminary data, described above, suggest that CBT-E may prove more effective than standard CBT for BN, perhaps because it is addressing personality features not adequately addressed in the original model and manual. Suggestive but highly preliminary research from our own laboratory suggests that most clinicians in the community attend closely to personality in EDs and employ integrative strategies to address both personality characteristics and target symptoms, and that these integrative approaches tend to yield better global and ED-specific outcomes than more 'pure' approaches. However, far more questions remain than have been addressed: How long is optimal treatment for ED patients with different forms of personality pathology? What is the best mix of symptom-focused versus diathesis-focused targets in therapy? What is the optimal timing of that mix (e.g. target symptoms first and personality diatheses once symptoms are under control, or target both simultaneously)? At this point, it would seem prudent for all treatment research on EDs to assess personality variables carefully as baseline predictors of outcome, as potential markers of likely response to various treatments (both pharmacological and psychotherapeutic), and as outcome variables.

Preparation of this article was supported in part by NIMH grants MH62377 and MH62378 to the first author.

Corresponding author: Drew Westen, Department of Psychology and Department of Psychiatry and Behavioral Sciences, Emory University, 532 Kilgo Circle, Atlanta, GA 30322, USA. Email: dwesten@emory.edu

References

References included from the targeted review years are preceded by one asterisk. References preceded by three asterisks are of particular significance. The significance is explained by a short commentary following the complete reference.

Agras WS, Crow SJ, Halmi KA, Mitchell JE, Wilson GT and Kraemer HC (2000) Outcome predictors for the cognitive behavior treatment of bulimia nervosa: Data from a multisite study. *American Journal of Psychiatry*, **157**: 1302–08.
*Anderluh MB, Tchanturia K, Rabe-Hesketh S and Treasure J (2003) Childhood obsessive-compulsive personality traits in adult women with EDs: Defining a broader ED phenotype. *American Journal of Psychiatry*, **160**: 242–7.

Bell L and Newns K (2002) What is multi-impulsive bulimia and can multi-impulsive patients benefit from supervised self-help? *European Eating Disorders Review*, **10(6)**: 413–27.

Bizeul C, Sadowsky N and Rigaud D (2001) The prognostic value of initial EDI scores in anorexia nervosa patients: a prospective follow-up study of 5–10 years. Eating Disorder Inventory. *European Psychiatry*, **16(4)**: 232–8.

*Bloks H, Hoek HW, Callewaert I and van Furth E (2004) Stability of personality traits in patients who received intensive treatment for a severe eating disorder. *Journal of Nervous and Mental Disease*, **192(2)**: 129–38.

Bossert S, Schmolz U, Wiegand M, Junker M and Krieg J (1992) Predictors of short-term treatment outcome in bulimia nervosa inpatients. *Behavior Research and Therapy*, **30**: 193–9.

Braun D, Sunday S and Halmi K (1994) Psychiatric comorbidity in patients with eating disorders. *Psychological Medicine*, **24**: 859–67.

***Bruce KR, Steiger H, Koerner NM, Israel M and Young SN (2004) Bulimia nervosa with co-morbid avoidant personality disorder: Behavioural characteristics and serotonergic function. *Psychological Medicine*, **34(1)**: 113–24.
This study was notable for the breadth of assessment measures converging on the finding of a consistently inhibited subtype of bulimia nervosa. In a sample with both BN and avoidant PD, the authors tested personality functioning (interpersonal inhibition and avoidance), neuropsychological functioning (errors of inhibition on the Go/No go task), and serotonergic functioning (deficits consistent with inhibited functioning). The study concludes that a distinct subtype exists, characterized by inhibition across three major domains.

Bulik C, Sullivan PF, Joyce PR, Carter FA and McIntosh VV (1998) Predictors of 1-year treatment outcome in bulimia nervosa. *Comprehensive Psychiatry*, **39**: 206–14.

*Bulik CM, Tozzi F, Anderson C, Mazzeo SE, Aggen S and Sullivan PF (2003) The relation between eating disorders and components of perfectionism. *American Journal of Psychiatry*, **160(2)**: 366–8.

*Cervera S, Lahortiga F, Martinez-Gonzalez MA, Gual P, Irala-Estevez J and Alonso Y (2003) Neuroticism and low self-esteem as risk factors for incident eating disorders in a prospective cohort study. *International Journal of Eating Disorders*, **33(3)**: 271–80.

Davis R, Olmsted MP and Rockert W (1992) Brief group psychoeducation for bulimia nervosa. II: Prediction of clinical outcome. *International Journal of Eating Disorders*, **11**: 205–11.

Eddy KT, Keel PK, Dorer DJ, Delinsky SS, Franko DL and Herzog DB (2002) Longitudinal comparison of AN subtypes. *International Journal of Eating Disorders*, **31(2)**: 191–201.

*Eddy K, Novotny C and Westen D (2004a) Sexuality, personality, and eating disorders. *Eating Disorders: The Journal of Treatment and Prevention*, **12**: 198–208.

*Eddy K, Thompson-Brenner H and Westen D (2004b) *Adolescent personality subtypes in patients with eating disorders*. Paper presented at the annual convention of the Academy for Eating Disorders, Orlando, Florida, April.

Espelage DL, Mazzeo SE, Sherman R and Thompson R (2002) MCMI-II profiles of women with eating disorders: A cluster analytic investigation. *Journal of Personality Disorders*, **16**: 453–63.

Fahy TA and Russell GFM (1993) Outcome and prognostic variables in bulimia nervosa. *International Journal of Eating Disorders*, **14**: 135–45.

***Fairburn CG (2004) *Keynote event: A dialogue about evidence-based practice*. Keynote Session at the Academy for Eating Disorders Annual Conference, Orlando, Florida, April.
This keynote address at the AED Annual Conference presented the first data regarding CBT-Enhanced, the new, flexible, transdiagnostic treatment for eating disorders. The presentation emphasized the point that empirically supported treatments exist only for

BN, whereas EDNOS is the most commonly diagnosed eating disorder in almost every clinical context. The presentation discussed the principles of CBT-E, including the 'focused' version that resembles earlier versions of CBT for BN but is tailored to the individual, the weight-gain version that is necessary for underweight patients, and the 'broad' version that can include modules addressing clinical perfectionism, mood intolerance, interpersonal problems, and low self-esteem. The first uncontrolled data for CBT-E suggested that over two-thirds of patients with EDNOS and BN recover by the end of treatment.

Fairburn CG, Peveler RC, Jones R, Hope RA and Doll HA (1993a) Predictors of 12-month outcome in bulimia nervosa and the influence of attitudes to shape and weight. *Journal of Consulting and Clinical Psychology*, **61**: 696–8.

Fairburn CG, Marcus MD and Wilson GT (1993b) Cognitive-behavioral therapy for binge eating and bulimia nervosa: A comprehensive treatment manual. In: CG Fairburn and GT Wilson (eds), *Binge Eating: nature, assessment and treatment*. Guilford Press, New York.

*Fairburn CG, Cooper Z and Shafran R (2003) Cognitive behaviour therapy for eating disorders: A 'transdiagnostic' theory and treatment. *Behaviour Research and Therapy*, **41**: 509–28.

*Fairburn CG, Bohn K and Hutt M (2004) *EDNOS (Eating Disorder not otherwise Specified): Why it is important, and how to treat it using cognitive behavior therapy*. Workshop Session at the Academy for Eating Disorders Annual Conference, Orlando, Florida, April.

Fassino S, Abbate DG, Amianto F, Leombruni P, Garzaro L and Rovera GG (2001) Nonresponder anorectic patients after 6 months of multimodal treatment: Predictors of outcome. *European Psychiatry*, **16(8)**: 466–73.

*Fassino S, Abbate-Daga G, Piero A, Leombruni P and Rovera GG (2003) Dropout from brief psychotherapy within a combination treatment in bulimia nervosa: Role of personality and anger. *Psychotherapy and Psychosomatics*, **72(4)**: 203–10.

*Fassino S, Amianto F, Gramaglia C, Facchini F and Abbate Daga G (2004) Temperament and character in eating disorders: Ten years of studies. *Eating and Weight Disorders*, **9(2)**: 81–90.

Fichter M, Quadflieg N and Rief W (1994) Course of multi-impulsive bulimia. *Psychological Medicine*, **24**: 591–604.

Ghaderi A and Scott B (2000) The Big Five and eating disorders: A prospective study in the general population. *European Journal of Personality*, **14**: 311–23.

Goldner EM, Srikameswaran S, Schroeder ML, Livesley WJ and Birmingham CL (1999) Dimensional assessment of personality pathology in patients with eating disorders. *Psychiatry Research*, **85**: 151–9.

*Grilo CM (2004) Subtyping female adolescent psychiatric inpatients with features of eating disorders along dietary restraint and negative affect dimensions. *Behaviour Research and Therapy*, **42(1)**: 67–78.

Grilo CM, Masheb RM and Berman RM (2001) Subtyping women with bulimia nervosa along dietary and negative affect dimensions: A replication in a treatment-seeking sample. *Eating and Weight Disorders*, **6**: 53–8.

*Grilo CM, Sanislow CA, Shea MT, Skodol AE, Stout RL, Pagano ME, Yen S and McGlashan TH (2003) The natural course of bulimia nervosa and eating disorder not otherwise specified is not influenced by personality disorders. *International Journal of Eating Disorders*, **34**: 319–30.

*Haas HL and Clopton JR (2003) Comparing clinical and research treatments for eating disorders. *International Journal of Eating Disorders*, **33**: 412–20.

*Halmi KA, Sunday SR, Klump KL, Strober M, Leckman JF, Fichter M, Kaplan A, Woodside B, Treasure J, Berrettini WH, Al Shabboat M, Bulik CM and Kaye WH (2003) Obsessions and compulsions in anorexia nervosa subtypes. *International Journal of Eating Disorders*, **33**: 308–19.

*Harnden-Fischer J, Thompson-Brenner H and Westen D (2005) *Emotional experience and emotion regulation in eating disorders*. Unpublished manuscript, Emory University, Georgia.

*Ilkjaer K, Kortegaard L, Hoerder K, Joergensen J, Kyvik K and Gillberg C (2004) Personality disorders in a total population twin cohort with eating disorders. *Comprehensive Psychiatry*, **45(4)**: 261–7.

Johnson C, Tobin DL and Dennis A (1990) Differences in treatment outcome between borderline and nonborderline bulimics at one-year follow-up. *International Journal of Eating Disorders*, **9**: 617–27.

*Kane TA, Loxton NJ, Staiger PK and Dawe S (2004) Does the tendency to act impulsively underlie binge eating and alcohol use problems? An empirical investigation. *Personality and Individual Differences*, **36**: 83–94.

*Kaye WH, Barbarich NC, Putnam K, Gendall KA, Fernstrom J, Fernstrom M, McConaha CW and Kishore A (2003) Anxiolytic effects of acute tryptophan depletion in anorexia nervosa. *International Journal of Eating Disorders*, **33(3)**: 257–67.

*Kendler KS, Prescott CA, Myers J and Neale MC (2003) The structure of genetic and environmental risk factors for common psychiatric and substance use disorders in men and women. *Archives of General Psychiatry*, **60(9)**: 929–37.

*Kotler LA, Boudreau GS and Devlin MJ (2003) Emerging psychotherapies for eating disorders. *Journal of Psychiatric Practice*, **9(6)**: 431–41.

Krueger RF (2002) The structure of common mental disorders. *Archives of General Psychiatry*, **59**: 570–1.

Lacey J and Evans C (1986) The impulsivist: A multi-impulsive personality disorder. *British Journal of Addiction*, **81**: 641–9.

Lilenfeld LRR, Wonderlich SA, Riso LPL, Crosby RD and Mitchell JE (in press) Eating disorders and personality: a methodological and empirical review. *Clinical Psychology Review*.

Linehan MM (1993) *Skills Training Manual for Treating Borderline Personality Disorder*. Guilford Press, New York.

Linehan MM, Cochran BN and Kehrer CA (2001) Dialectical behavior therapy for borderline personality disorder. In: DH Barlow (ed), *Clinical Handbook of Psychological Disorders: a step-by-step treatment manual*. Guilford Press, New York, pp 470–522.

*Markon KE, Krueger RF and Watson D (2005) Delineating the structure of normal and abnormal personality: An integrative hierarchical approach. *Journal of Personality and Social Psychology*, **88**: 139–57.

Matsunaga H, Kiriike N, Iwasaki Y, Miyata A, Matsui T, Nagata T, Yamagami S and Kaye WH (2000) Multi-impulsivity among bulimic patients in Japan. *International Journal of Eating Disorders*, **27(3)**: 348–52.

McMain S, Korman LM and Dimeff L (2001) Dialectical behavior therapy and the treatment of emotional dysregulation. *Journal of Clinical Psychology*, **57**: 183–96.

*Milos G, Spindler AM, Buddeberg C and Crameri A (2003) Axes I and II comorbidity and treatment experiences in eating disorder subjects. *Psychotherapy and Psychosomatics*, **72(5)**: 276–85.

*Milos G, Spindler A and Schnyder U (2004) Psychiatric comorbidity and Eating Disorder Inventory (EDI) profiles in eating disorder patients. *Canadian Journal of Psychiatry*, **49(3)**: 179–84.

*Nagata T, Oshima J, Wada A, Yamada H, Iketani T and Kiriike N (2003) Temperament and character of Japanese eating disorder patients. *Comprehensive Psychiatry*, **44(2)**: 142–5.

*Palmer RL, Birchall H, Damani S, Gatward N, McGrain L and Parker L (2003) A dialectical behavior therapy program for people with an eating disorder and borderline personality disorder–description and outcome. *International Journal of Eating Disorders*, **33**: 281–6.

*Perkins PS, Klump KL, Iacono WG and McGue M (2005) Personality traits in women with anorexia nervosa: evidence for a treatment-seeking bias? *International Journal of Eating Disorders*, **37(1)**: 32–7.

*Rastam M, Gillberg C and Wentz E (2003) Outcome of teenage-onset anorexia nervosa in a Swedish community-based sample. *European and Child Adolescent Psychiatry*, **12**: I78–90.

Robins E and S Guze (1970) The establishment of diagnostic validity in psychiatric illness: its application to schizophrenia. *American Journal of Psychiatry*, **126**: 983–7.

Rossiter EM, Agras WS, Telch CF and Schneider JA (1993) Cluster B personality disorder characteristics predict outcome in the treatment of bulimia nervosa. *International Journal of Eating Disorders*, **13**: 349–57.

Safer DL, Telch CF and Agras WS (2001) Dialectical behavior therapy for bulimia nervosa. *American Journal of Psychiatry*, **158**: 632–4.

*Sherry SB, Hewitt PL, Besser A, McGee BJ and Flett G (2004) Self-oriented and socially prescribed perfectionism in the Eating Disorder Inventory Perfectionism Subscale. *International Journal of Eating Disorders*, **35**: 69–79.

Skodol A, Oldham J, Hyler S, Kellman H, Doidge N and Davies M (1993) Comorbidity of DSM-III-R eating disorders and personality disorders. *International Journal of Eating Disorders*, **14**: 403–16.

Steiger H and Stotland S (1996) Prospective study of outcome in bulimics as a function of axis-II comorbidity: Long-term responses on eating and psychiatric symptoms. *International Journal of Eating Disorders*, **20**: 149–61.

*Steiger H, Israel M, Gauvin L, Ng Ying Kin NM and Young SN (2003) Implications of compulsive and impulsive traits for serotonin status in women with bulimia nervosa. *Psychiatry Research*, **120(3)**: 219–29.

*Steiger H, Gauvin L, Israel M, Kin NM, Young SN and Roussin J (2004) Serotonin function, personality-trait variations, and childhood abuse in women with bulimia-spectrum eating disorders. *Journal of Clinical Psychiatry*, **65**: 830–7.

Steinhausen HC (2002) The outcome of anorexia nervosa in the 20th century. *American Journal of Psychiatry*, **159(8)**: 1284–93.

Stice E (2002) Risk and maintenance factors for eating pathology: A meta-analytic review. *Psychological Bulletin*, **128(5)**: 825–48.

Stice E and Agras WS (1999) Subtyping women along dietary restraint and negative affect dimensions. *Journal of Consulting and Clinical Psychology*, **67**: 460–9.

*Stice E and Fairburn CG (2003) Dietary and dietary-depressive subtypes of bulimia nervosa show differential symptom presentation, social impairment, comorbidity, and course of illness. *Journal of Consulting and Clinical Psychology*, **71**: 1090–4.

*Stice E, Peart J, Thompson-Brenner H, Martinez E and Westen D (in press) Eating disorders. In: F Andrasik (ed), *The Comprehensive Handbook of Personality and Psychopathology: Volume II: adult psychopathology*. Wiley, Hoboken, NJ.

*Sutandar-Pinnock K, Blake Woodside D, Carter JC, Olmsted MP and Kaplan AS (2003) Perfectionism in anorexia nervosa: a 6–24-month follow-up study. *International Journal of Eating Disorders*, **33(2)**: 225–9.

Telch CF, Agras WS and Linehan MM (2000) Group dialectical behavior therapy for binge-eating disorder: A preliminary, uncontrolled trial. *Behavior Therapy*, **31**: 569–75.

Telch CF, Agras WS and Linehan MM (2001) Dialectical behavior therapy for binge eating disorder. *Journal of Consulting and Clinical Psychology*, **69**: 1061–5.

*Thompson-Brenner H and Westen D (2005a) A naturalistic study of treatment for bulimia, Part 1: Comorbidity and therapeutic outcome. *Journal of Nervous and Mental Disease*, **193(9)**: 573–84.

***Thompson-Brenner H and Westen D (2005b) A naturalistic study of treatment for bulimia, Part 2: Therapeutic interventions in the community. *Journal of Nervous and Mental Disease*, **193(9)**: 585–95.

This two-part article presents data from a clinician-report study of 145 patients with bulimic pathology treated in the community. Results from the community support prior observations that rates of comorbidity are very high and are related to treatment outcome. Results supported the observation of three personality subtypes, with treatment length and outcome associated with subtype. The use of cognitive-behavioral interventions was associated with more rapid remission, whereas the use of psychodynamic interventions was associated with global outcome.

*Thompson-Brenner H and Westen D (2005c) Personality subtypes in eating disorders: Validation of a classification in a naturalistic sample. *British Journal of Psychiatry*, **186**: 516–24.

*Thompson-Brenner H, Glass S and Westen D (2003) A multidimensional meta-analysis of psychotherapy for bulimia nervosa. *Clinical Psychology: Research and Practice*, **10(3)**: 269–87.

*Vervaet M, van Heeringen C and Audenaert K (2004) Personality-related characteristics in restricting versus binging and purging eating disordered patients. *Comprehensive Psychiatry*, **45(1)**: 37–43.

Vitousek K and Manke F (1994) Personality variables and disorders in anorexia nervosa and bulimia nervosa. *Journal of Abnormal Psychology*, **103**: 137–47.

Westen D (1997) Divergences between clinical and research methods for assessing personality disorders: Implications for research and the evolution of Axis II. *American Journal of Psychiatry*, **154**: 895–903.

Westen D and Harnden-Fischer J (2001) Personality profiles in eating disorders: Rethinking the distinction between axis I and axis II. *American Journal of Psychiatry*, **158**: 547–62.

*Westen D, Gabbard G and Blagov P (in press) Back to the future: Personality structure as a context for psychopathology. In: RF Krueger and JL Tackett (eds), *Personality and Psychopathology*. Guilford Press, New York.

*Wisniewski L and Kelly E (2003) The application of dialectical behavior therapy to the treatment of eating disorders. *Cognitive and Behavioral Practice*, **10**: 131–8.

Wonderlich SA, Fullerton D, Swift WJ and Klein MH (1994) Five-year outcome from eating disorders: Relevance of personality disorders. *International Journal of Eating Disorders*, **15**: 233–43.

***Wonderlich SA, Connolly KM and Stice E (2004) Impulsivity as a risk factor for eating disorder behavior: Assessment implications with adolescents. *International Journal of Eating Disorders*, **36**: 172–82.

This study investigated the role of impulsivity as a risk factor for disordered eating. The primary goal was to establish whether risk outcomes depended on the way that impulsivity was measured. The researchers found that trait impulsivity, as measured by traditional personality scales, failed to predict the onset of eating pathology. However, behavioral indicators of impulsivity, such as substance abuse or delinquency, significantly predicted the onset of disordered eating.

***Wonderlich SA, Crosby RD, Joiner T, Peterson CB, Bardone-Cone A, Klein M, Crow S, Mitchell JE, le Grange D, Steiger H, Kolden G, Johnson F and Vrshek S (2005a) Personality subtyping and bulimia nervosa: Psychopathological and genetic correlates. *Psychological Medicine*, **35(5)**: 649–57.

This multi-site study combined data on 178 patients with clinical or sub-clinical BN, including data on ED symptoms, personality pathology, perfectionism, impulsivity,

drug abuse, depression, anxiety, obsessive–compulsive behavior, and genetic information. Latent profile analysis including the variables above (excluding ED symptoms) produced a stable three-cluster solution. Clusters were labeled 'High-functioning', 'Affective–Perfectionistic', and 'Impulsive'. The affective–perfectionistic cluster had significantly higher scores on perfectionism, obsessive–compulsive symptoms, trait anxiety, inhibitedness, and depression. The impulsive cluster had significantly higher scores on impulsive/self-destructive behavior, dissocial behavior, and substance abuse.

***Wonderlich SA, Lilenfeld LR, Riso LP, Engel S and Mitchell JE (2005b) Personality and anorexia nervosa. *International Journal of Eating Disorders*, **37(S1)**: S68–S71.

This article reviews the extant literature on eating disorders and anorexia nervosa. The major conceptual models of the relationship between personality and anorexia nervosa are reviewed. In addition, the authors review methodological challenges for eating disorder and personality research and suggest more clarity in the conceptual models that researchers apply to their future work.

*Zanarini MC, Frankenburg FR, Hennen J, Reich DB and Silk KR (2004) Axis I comorbidity in patients with borderline personality disorder: 6-year follow-up and prediction of time to remission. *American Journal of Psychiatry*, **161(11)**: 2108–14.

7

Review of brain imaging in anorexia and bulimia nervosa

*Walter H Kaye, Angela Wagner, Guido Frank
and Ursula F Bailer*

Abstract

Objectives of review. Advances in brain imaging provide new understanding of how brain regions and neurotransmitter circuits may be related to appetitive dysregulation, mood problems, obsessionality, and body image distortions in anorexia and bulimia nervosa (AN and BN)

Summary of recent findings. Imaging studies in healthy humans have characterized brain regions such as the insula, anterior cingulate, and orbital frontal cortex that modulate higher order appetitive behaviors. Studies using food-related stimuli raise the possibility of altered function of such regions in AN and BN. Other imaging studies have confirmed that alterations of serotonin occur in the ill state and after recovery from AN and BN, supporting the possibility that disturbed serotonin function may be a trait. Moreover, imaging studies have begun to identify how serotonin receptors and the transporter function are related to potential behavioral traits, such as anxiety. Several recent studies find alterations of L parietal function may be related to body image distortion, offering new insights into this most puzzling symptom.

Future directions. It is likely that imaging will be of major importance in identifying brain regions and neurocircuits that may be related to altered appetite, mood, impulse control, body image, and other symptoms of AN and BN. Such understandings may help to destigmatize AN and BN and contribute to better treatment.

Introduction

There is growing acknowledgment that neurobiological vulnerabilities make a substantial contribution to the pathogenesis of AN and BN. Still, we have little understanding of how such vulnerabilities result in disturbances of brain pathways or what systems are primarily involved. For example, are there disturbances of pathways related to the modulation of feeding behaviors, or mood, or temperament, or obsessionality, or impulse control? Are there primary disturbances of pathways that may modulate some factors related to body proprioception, and thus result in body-image distortions? The past decade has seen the introduction of tools, such as brain imaging, which hold the promise of being able to characterize complex neurocircuits and their relationship to behavior, in living humans. In fact, these tools have rapidly advanced knowledge to the point where we can begin to make educated guesses about the pathophysiology of AN and BN and start to model mechanisms that may be used to test hypotheses.

Brain-imaging studies in AN and BN can be divided into several categories. First, there has been substantial literature, using CT and more recently MRI, which seeks to determine whether there are brain structural alterations in individuals with EDs. Second, more recent studies have used functional magnetic resonance imaging (fMRI) or other technologies to assess blood flow responses to some stimuli, such as pictures of food. Third are imaging studies, such as PET and SPECT, which employ a radioligand. These studies, which may use flurodeoxyglucose (FDG) to study glucose metabolism or a ligand that is specific for a serotonin receptor, provide information that is specific for the system being studied, such as the 5-HT$_{2A}$ receptor.

In general, imaging studies have been relatively consistent, in that most studies have findings in frontal, cingulate, temporal, and/or parietal regions. Thus it can be stated that individuals with EDs, when ill and after recovery, have alterations in brain activity compared to matched controls. However, it should be noted that these studies have not consistently identified regions, pathways, or behavioral correlates. Sample sizes have been small, and imaging technologies and methods vary widely. Moreover, investigations have tended to assess relatively large regions of brain that vary widely between studies. Moreover, papers to date indicate gross alterations of brain function. Because brain pathways are highly complex, the neuroanatomy of AN and BN has only begun to be characterized.

It should be noted that there has been substantial progress in understanding how brain cortical regions modulate higher order functions related to appetitive behaviors in humans. Thus this review begins with an overview of this work, since it provides a potential baseline that can be used to determine whether individuals with AN and BN have some alteration in brain pathways devoted to the modulation of feeding.

Review of imaging studies of normal feeding behavior in healthy individuals

Overview

Before discussing findings from brain-imaging studies in individuals with AN and BN, we review recent literature on feeding-related physiology in healthy controls. The system of appetite and hunger, food appetence, ingestion of food and subsequent subjective experience is very complex and study methodologies and results are not homogeneous. However, those studies may help us guide research on the pathophysiology of EDs and delineate biological traits. Little work has been done in AN and BN in understanding how taste and olfaction might activate brain circuits. Perhaps the primary question is whether individuals with AN or BN have alterations of feeding-related brain pathways and how phenomena such as food-related anxiety play a role in the physiology of ED.

Review of studies in the past two years

Recent studies have shown that it is possible to study taste and smell in conjunction with fMRI which may inform studies in the ED population (De Araujo *et al*. 2003; Cerf-Ducastel and Murphy 2004). In brief, the insula cortex shows the primary response to taste recognition and the orbitofrontal cortex (OFC) shows secondary response to various taste stimuli. Stimuli such as pleasant taste activate the OFC. This activation declines when the same food is presented repeatedly which is called sensory-specific satiety. New studies now show that the dorsolateral prefrontal cortex is responsive to gustatory activation (Kringelbach *et al*. 2004). This area is a cognitive processing center and may suggest cognitive reflection of the taste experience, perhaps on a tertiary level. In a review of their own and studies of other investigators, this group proposes that the OFC activity may be separated into anterior–posterior and medial–lateral compartments with task-specific responsiveness (Kringelbach *et al*. 2004). With the notion that the OFC is involved in the evaluation of the reward value that a stimulus has, the medial part may then be active to reinforcing and the lateral part to aversive stimuli. This may also be the case for olfactory stimuli (Gottfried *et al*. 2002). The anterior part was hypothesized to be more involved in abstract stimuli such as monetary reward as opposed to more primitive experiences including taste or pain.

Another recent study commented on the interaction between the OFC and the amygdala (Arana *et al*. 2003). Using a paradigm where subjects had to select food items from different menus, it was found that the amygdala responded relative to the appeal of the food on the menu. The medial OFC, however, was activated when having to make choices between menu items and this brain response correlated with the individual's subjectively perceived difficulty during that task. The lateral OFC was activated when the preferred menu could not be chosen.

These studies suggest testable hypotheses for understanding AN and BN. Individuals with restricting type AN may have higher lateral OFC activation to aversive and perhaps anxiety-provoking food stimuli such as fat (Drewnowski *et al.* 1987b) but higher medial OFC activity in response to exercise, weight loss-promoting activity or particularly 'safe' foods. It is also possible that individuals with AN have a quick onset of sensory-specific satiety, which could be related to an accelerated reduction of OFC response to food stimuli, thus resulting in early meal termination. Individuals with BN, in contrast, may have a delayed medial OFC activation reduction (delayed sensory specific satiety), resulting in over-eating. Although BN patients may like sweeter stimuli than controls (Drewnowski *et al.* 1987a), they may have increased medial OFC response, but they may also have increased amygdala activation, perhaps related to heightened anxiety after binge-eating episodes. It is important to note that humans have substantial variability of brain response to taste stimuli, which may limit the power and interpretability of study results (Schoenfeld *et al.* 2004).

As noted below, brain-imaging studies in individuals with EDs have used pictures of food and similar food-related stimuli to investigate appetite regulation. Recent studies in controls confirmed that pictures of food activate primary and secondary taste centers as well as other regions (Wang *et al.* 2004). In another study, both high- and low-calorie food images activated the amygdala and ventromedial prefrontral cortex. However, high-calorie foods may stimulate more medial and dorsolateral prefrontal areas, whereas low-calorie food images may activate medial OFC and temporal regions (Killgore *et al.* 2003). Brain-imaging studies using pictures of food test motivational states and possibly the desire to approach food. The hunger state in fact seems to activate the amygdala and temporal areas more than the satiation state (LaBar *et al.* 2001) although sex differences seem to exist. It would be of interest to determine whether there is an appetitive difference in ED subjects and if AN subjects are more resilient toward hunger. Other important questions include whether individuals with AN ignore hunger because of heightened anxiety when considering possible weight gain and if brain response such as ACC or amygdala activity associated with anxiety ratings could reflect such altered processing of hunger and a desire to eat.

Little work has been done assessing neurochemical alterations involved in the feeding network. One study, using PET and the dopamine (DA) D2/D3 radio-ligand raclopride, found lower raclopride binding in the dorsal putamen and caudate nucleus in the satiated state compared to a hunger state, suggesting DA release during or after the feeding process. In addition, the experienced meal pleasantness correlated negatively with raclopride binding, suggesting a positive correlation of pleasantness rating with DA surge (Small *et al.* 2003). This is surprising since in many studies pleasantness or hedonic experiences were related to DA activity in the ventral striatum, including the nucleus accumbens. Studying neuroreceptor networks is of particular importance since results may contribute to developing new pharmaceutical interventions. The DA system may be of particular interest because it plays a role in motivation, reward, preferences and reinforcement (Cannon and Bseikri 2004).

Another interesting study was on taste and preconceptions about the food ingested, suggesting that what we think about a certain product may be more influential than the substance itself when we cannot distinguish the taste (McClure *et al.* 2004). This is a highly important issue for individuals with EDs, who experience aversiveness in response to food based on its presumed calorie content rather than taste itself.

AN and BN primarily occur in women. A recent study showed differences between sexes in response to a liquid meal during hunger or satiation state (Del Parigi *et al.* 2002). In particular, women had higher activity in occipital and parietal sensory association cortex and in the dorsolateral prefrontal cortex, but men had greater activation in the ventromedial prefrontal cortex when satiated. This study did not report on other behavioral/emotional parameters, but it is possible that there are gender differences in terms of response to food items and taste. However, this is speculative and needs to be further tested. A design that investigates the cognitive impact versus a more basic physiologic processing in women versus men and then in ED subjects should be pursued. Furthermore, it would be very interesting to assess similarities and differences between women versus men who all have AN or BN.

In summary, the study of normal brain activity in relation to food intake has identified cortical pathways related to the physiology of food intake, such as the insula. In particular, the medial OFC may be somewhat specific for pleasant, and the lateral OFC specific for aversive taste experiences. In addition, the prefrontal cortex may be involved in cognitive processing of the food ingestion. In this network of activation, the amygdala was confirmed to play a role and may respond relative to the incentive and emotional value of taste stimulus. The balance between learned behaviors and innate biological traits is not certain, since knowledge about the brand name of a taste stimulus may contribute to brain activation. Studies have used tastes of food and food images in controls. However, little work has been done in determining whether brain responses are similar using different types of food-related stimuli. This may be of importance in understanding cognitive influences of taste. Also interesting are data suggesting that men and women have different responses to food as, for example, the possibility that women have greater cognitive activation to food stimuli as well as sensorimotor cortex activation in response to a liquid meal after satiation. Such studies may shed light on understanding why women are at greater risk of developing EDs. Of importance is new understanding of DA and the hedonics of appetite regulation since the DA system may be altered in AN. Together these studies offer important new leads for the study of altered eating physiology in AN and BN.

fMRI and task activation studies

Overview

A number of studies have used fMRI and single photon emission computed tomography (SPECT) to investigate appetite regulation in AN and BN. In general, sample sizes have been small, and studies have used a range of methods and explored many different brain regions. Moreover, the resolution of SPECT is poor so that specific regions cannot be clearly identified. While many of the studies have found alterations in brain response, there have been few attempts to replicate findings. In brief, Nozoe measured regional cerebral blood flow (rCBF) using SPECT and detected a significant increase in response to food intake in the left inferior frontal cortex in AN compared to controls (Nozoe et al. 1993). In a later study Nozoe (Nozoe et al. 1995) reported that individuals with AN did not have cortical laterality or activated state in any cortical area before eating. However, there was increased activity in frontal, occipital, parietal and temporal regions after eating. In contrast, BN showed the highest cortical activity in the left temporal region and the bilateral inferior frontal regions before eating compared to controls but less cortical activity in response to food intake. Naruo (Naruo et al. 2000) reported that food imagination assessed by SPECT results in greater activation in inferior, superior, prefrontal and parietal regions of the right brain in binge/purge type AN in comparison to restricting type AN and healthy controls. Gordon et al. (2001) used PET to show that a high-calorie food stimulus resulted in elevated rCBF in occipital temporal regions in individuals with AN compared to controls. Ellison et al. (1998) used fMRI and found that individuals with AN, when viewing pictures of high-calorie drinks, had increased signal changes in the left insula, anterior cingulate cortex and left amygdala-hippocampal region that were possibly anxiety related. The amygdala-hippocampus region was also activated in healthy volunteers when confronted with unpleasant words concerning body image relative to neutral words and negatively correlated to parts of the Eating Disorder Inventory-2 (Shirao et al. 2003). In addition, a decrease of blood flow in the anterior cingulate region was detected by Takano using SPECT in AN compared to controls. In summary, the many positive findings suggested the importance of proceeding with new brain-imaging studies of appetite regulation, but a need to localize regions, identify neural circuits, replicate findings, and link results to other human and animal literature.

Review of fMRI studies in the past two years

Uher and colleagues assessed 26 female ED patients (16 AN, 10 BN) and compared them to 19 age-matched controls using fMRI (Uher et al. 2004). During scanning subjects were confronted with images of food and nonfood items as well as emotional aversive and neutral images. In response to food stimuli, AN subjects, in comparison to controls, had higher activation in the left medial orbitofrontal and anterior cingulate cortex and a lower activation in the lateral prefrontal cortex, inferior parietal lobule and cerebellum. BN showed less activation in the lateral prefrontal cortex relative to controls for this stimulus. In contrast, the group contrast for the emotional stimuli reveals significant activation in the occipital cortex, parietal cortex and cerebellum. It is important to note that Uher et al. (2004) included ill subjects (n=8) previously described in an earlier paper (Uher et al. 2003). In the former study the authors found that eight ill subjects, when compared to nine restricting-type AN, had increased right lateral and apical prefrontal cortex and anterior cingulate cortex activation in response to food stimuli. Still, recovered AN subjects showed increased medial prefrontal and anterior cingulate activation as well as decreased inferior parietal lobule activation to food stimuli in comparison to healthy controls. In this study neural processing of emotional stimuli did not differ between groups. This is an important study for several reasons. First, it is the largest sample of ED patients studied with fMRI to date. Second, it compared stimuli related to food and emotions. These findings suggest that the medial prefrontal cortex might be specifically related to food stimuli since other regions were activated by both food and emotional stimuli. Activation of the lateral prefrontal cortex might be related to good outcome as it differentiated ill and recovered subjects. In general, findings are largely compatible with previous reports in subjects with EDs except for the lack of an amygdala activation in the large sample, which could be related to methodological issues.

Wagner and colleagues confronted 13 AN patients and 10 age-matched healthy controls with their own digitally distorted body images as well as images of a different person using a computer-based video technique (Seeger *et al.* 2002; Wagner *et al.* 2003). These studies reported a hyper-responsiveness in brain areas belonging to the frontal visual system and the attention network (BA 9) as well as inferior parietal lobule (BA 40), including the anterior part of the intraparietal (IPL) sulcus. However, an analysis of the 'blood oxygen level Dependent' response in the IPL area revealed that AN showed only a specific increase in activation to their own pictures rather than to others, indicating different visuo-spatial processing, while controls did not differentiate. Perceptual alterations might be related to the neglect phenomenon. The authors did not replicate amygdala activation as found in a pilot study of three AN subjects (Seeger *et al.* 2002). This is the first study using a visual challenge of their own body and fMRI to assess body-image distortion in AN. The identified brain regions are consistent with findings in PET, which also associated these areas with body-image distortion (Bailer *et al.* 2004b) as described below. It would be interesting to repeat this paradigm with recovered subjects to detect whether this symptom persists after recovery.

Our group (Frank *et al.* 2003) reported on new methodology developed to determine whether individuals with AN and BN have altered brain physiological response to macronutrients, such as sugars. In this paradigm, glucose and artificial saliva are administered blindly by a programmable syringe pump that coordinates taste stimulation with fMRI scanning. Five healthy women showed increased OFC activation when glucose was delivered compared to artificial saliva. In addition, mesial and lateral temporal cortical regions contrasted glucose from artificial saliva. Applying this paradigm to 10 recovered BN and six control women (CW), the recovered subjects had a significantly lower activation in the right anterior cingulate cortex and left cuneus when both stimuli were compared (Frank *et al.* 2002a). These findings suggest a reduced reward response to nutrients in BN.

Wagner further developed the paradigm to assess habituation effects to repeated taste experiences. For this purpose 10% sucrose solution and distilled water were either administered repeatedly and sequentially or pseudo-randomly alternated to 11 healthy female subjects while undergoing fMRI (Wagner *et al.* 2004). To test habituation, activation during the first half of each block was compared to activation during the second half of each block. Regions of interest (ROI) included the insula, OFC, dorsolateral prefrontal cortex and amygdala. For the pseudo-random blocks, subjects showed habituation to water in all ROIs, but no ROI showed habituation to sucrose. However, for sequential blocks, both water and sucrose showed habituation for all ROIs. These data suggest that habituation patterns in healthy subjects may be related to methods of stimulus administration.

In summary, several laboratories are developing studies using fMRI that have the potential of understanding brain neurocircuitry that may contribute to phenomena such as appetite dysregulation and body-image distortions in AN and BN.

Structural brain alterations

Overview

Postmortem studies in individuals who were ill with AN have demonstrated reduced cerebral mass with prominent sulci and small gyri (Gagel 1953; Martin 1958). Neuroimaging studies with CT reported cerebral atrophy and enlarged ventricles in ill AN (Heinz *et al.* 1977; Nussbaum *et al.* 1980; Zeumer *et al.* 1982; Kohlmeyer *et al.* 1983; Artmann *et al.* 1985; Lankenau *et al.* 1985; Dolan *et al.* 1988; Krieg *et al.* 1988; Palazidou *et al.* 1990). In BN, similar but less pronounced structural brain abnormalities were reported (Krieg *et al.* 1989) and may have been related to a chronic dietary restriction. More recently, MRI studies in AN showed larger cerebrospinal fluid (CSF) volumes in association with deficits in both total gray matter (GM) and total white matter (WM) volumes (Katzman *et al.* 1996) as well as enlarged ventricles (Kronreich *et al.* 1991; Golden *et al.* 1996; Swayze *et al.* 1996). Fewer neuroimaging studies have been conducted in BN, and those have found decreased cortical mass (Laessle *et al.* 1989; Hoffman 1989; Husain 1992).

Limited investigations have been done on more or less weight-restored subjects. They consistently report a decrease of the enlarged ventricles after weight gain in AN (Golden *et al.* 1996; Kingston *et al.* 1996; Swayze *et al.* 1996). Lambe found an increase in gray and white matter volumes as well as a decrease in CSF volume in recovered AN in comparison to ill AN subjects. Compared to control women, recovered AN had greater CSF volume and smaller GM, but showed no WM volume deficits. The recovered subjects were weight restored for at least one year and had started to menstruate or returned to normal menses at the time of follow-up (Lambe *et al.* 1997). Katzman replicated these findings in a longitudinal study of a subset of six weight-recovered subjects with a history of AN (Katzman *et al.* 1997). More recently Neumarker *et al.* (2000) compared ANs with controls and did follow-ups after 50% weight restoration and after achieving normal weight. AN subjects showed a significant volume difference of the lateral ventricles and the fissure of Sylvius which abated with weight restoration, whereas deficits of the mesencephalon and pons persisted (Neumarker *et al.* 2000).

Studies in the last two years

Swayze examined 17 AN patients as well as 18 sex- and age-matched and height-equivalent controls (Swayze *et al.* 2003). Thirteen of the AN had a follow-up scan after weight normalization at a mean of 107 days after the initial scan. Total and regional WM volume were significantly reduced and total and regional CSF volumes were significantly increased in ill AN subjects compared to controls. However, GM was not significantly reduced compared to controls. All three tissue volumes were different in the parietal lobes. After weight normalization, AN subjects had total and regional CSF volumes that were significantly decreased whereas WM and GM volumes were increased compared to the ill state. A strength of this study is that the authors looked also for regional differences. Unfortunately, the follow-up scan was not compared to the control subjects, although subjects were assessed longitudinally. In addition, subjects were not fully recovered–rather they were just weight-restored subjects. No information was reported on length of weight normalization or other criteria of recovery such as, for example, menses status.

Taken together, the studies report atrophy in ill AN subjects with reduced GM and WM volumes as well as increased CSF volumes. However, it is less clear whether recovery leads to partial or full reversibility of those brain abnormalities. Most studies lack a sufficient sample size, a rigid definition of recovery or a comparison of the findings with control subjects which should be addressed in future investigations.

Brain-imaging studies of neurotransmitter function

Overview

Brain imaging with radioligands offers the possibility of better understanding of serotonin (5-HT) neurotransmitter activity and dynamic relationships to behavior. Technologies used to date include SPECT and PET studies. Differences in resolution of imaging technologies, radioligands, characteristics of subject groups, and ROIs make it difficult to directly compare studies in terms of brain pathways involved. Still, these studies tend to have consistent findings as has been shown in publications from different laboratories in the last two years.

Studies in the last two years

Studies from our group have used PET with [^{18}F]altanserin binding potential (BP) to characterize the 5-HT$_{2A}$ receptor. This receptor is of interest because it has been implicated in the regulation of feeding, mood, and anxiety, and in antidepressant action (Barnes and Sharp 1999). Our group (Frank *et al.* 2002a,b; Bailer *et al.* 2004a) has found that both recovered (REC) AN and AN–BN have reduced [^{18}F]altanserin BP in the subgenual cingulate, parietal, and occipital cortex. In addition, REC AN had reduced [^{18}F]altanserin BP of the mesial temporal region and pregenual cingulate (Frank *et al.* 2002b), while REC BN showed a decrease of [^{18}F]altanserin BP only in the medial orbital frontal cortex (Kaye *et al.* 2001). Other studies of ill, underweight AN, which used SPECT with a 5-HT$_{2A}$ receptor antagonist (Audenaert *et al.* 2003), found a significant reduction of 5-HT$_{2A}$ receptor activity in the left frontal cortex, the left and right parietal cortex, and the left and right occipital cortex. However, it is not clear whether ill AN subjects were pure restrictors or included any AN-BN subtypes. Still, these studies are consistent in terms of reporting reduced 5-HT$_{2A}$ activity in cortical regions in AN, and findings seem to be independent of state of illness.

A further important step in these technologies is to correlate the assessed 5-HT activity with behavior. Bailer *et al.* (2004b) found that REC AN–BN subjects showed a positive relationship between [^{18}F]altanserin BP in the left subgenual cingulate and mesial temporal cortex and harm avoidance. Furthermore, negative relationships between novelty seeking and [^{18}F]altanserin BP were found in REC AN–BN in the left subgenual cingulate, the pregenual cingulate, and mesial temporal cortex. The AN studies described above (Frank *et al.* 2002b; Audenaert *et al.* 2003; Bailer *et al.* 2004a) have all found alterations in 5HT$_{2A}$ activity in the left parietal region. Furthermore, Bailer *et al.* (2004a) found negative relationships between [^{18}F]altanserin BP and a measure of drive for thinness in several regions including the left parietal cortex. A core symptom in AN is the relentless pursuit of thinness and obsessive fear of being fat. These findings raise the speculation that left parietal alterations in REC AN and AN–BN might contribute to body-image distortions, as suggested also by other groups, using fMRI (Wagner *et al.* 2003). To our knowledge no other studies have reported relationships between 5HT$_{2A}$ binding and behavior in individuals with ED so far.

Several groups have assessed the 5-HT$_{1A}$ receptor in AN, as this receptor may play a role in anxiety, mood and impulse control, feeding behavior, as well as in SSRI response. Our group has used PET imaging with the radioligand [^{11}C]WAY100635 to assess pre- and postsynaptic 5-HT$_{1A}$ receptor function in AN. We found that REC AN–BN (Bailer *et al.* 2004a) had increased [^{11}C]WAY100635 BP in prefrontal, lateral and medial orbital frontal, lateral temporal, parietal, supra- and pregenual cingulate regions as well as in the dorsal raphe, after adjustment for multiple comparisons. REC restricting-type anorexia nervosa (RAN) did not differ significantly from matched CW in any of the assessed regions. Only REC RAN had positive relationships between harm avoidance and postsynaptic [^{11}C]WAY100635 BP in subgenual cingulate, mesial temporal, lateral temporal, medial orbital frontal, and parietal cortex. Such correlations were not found in REC BAN subjects.

It is of much interest that other studies from our group (Bailer *et al.* 2004b) found that REC BAN had positive relationships between harm avoidance and [^{18}F]altanserin BP in the left subgenual cingulate, left lateral temporal and mesial temporal cortex. Such relationships were not found in REC RAN (Frank *et al.* 2002b). Together, these studies raise the possibility that cingulate and temporal regions may play a role in elevated harm avoidance in people with EDs.

Several lines of evidence support the possibility that disturbances of DA function could contribute to alterations of weight, feeding, motor activity, and reward in AN. Our group used PET with [^{11}C]raclopride to assess DA D2/D3 receptor binding in 10 REC AN compared to 12 healthy controls (Kaye *et al.* 2004). REC AN had significantly higher [^{11}C]raclopride BP in the antero-ventral striatum. These data lend support for the possibility that decreased intrasynaptic DA concentrations or increased D2/D3 receptor density or affinity are associated with AN, and may contribute to the characteristic increased physical activity found in AN. In terms of limitations, this pilot study combined restricting- and binge-purge type REC AN in order to increase sample size. Future studies with larger sample sizes will have to determine whether there are subgroup differences in AN.

There are only a few studies undertaken in BN so far and the results are less consistent compared to the more robust findings in AN. Ill BN have been found to have normal 5-HT$_{2A}$ receptor activity (Goethals *et al.* 2004) while REC BN have reduced [^{18}F]altanserin BP in the medial orbital frontal cortex (Kaye *et al.* 2001). Tauscher *et al.* (2001) found a reduction in 5-HT transporter availability in the thalamus and hypothalamus in 10 women who were ill with BN using SPECT with [^{123}I]-2beta-carbomethoxy-3beta-(4-iodophenyl) tropane. It should be noted that sample sizes are relatively small. Moreover, investigators have concentrated on assessment of different regions, and imaging techniques vary in terms of resolution.

Preliminary data in REC BN (Kaye *et al.* 2004) have also found increased [^{11}C]WAY100635 BP throughout the cortex and in the raphe. In support of the possibility of alterations in 5-HT$_{1A}$ activity and associated pathways in BN, increased postsynaptic 5-HT$_{1A}$ activity has been reported in ill BN subjects (Tiihonen *et al.* 2004) using PET and [^{11}C]WAY100635. Ill BN had increased [^{11}C]WAY100635 in frontal, cingulate, temporal, and raphe regions. The most robust differences were observed in the angular gyrus, the medial prefrontal cortex, and the posterior cingulate cortex.

Taken together, the studies described above raise the possibility that anorexic subtypes may share a disturbance of 5-HT$_{2A}$ receptor activity of the subgenual cingulate, whereas regional differences in 5-HT$_{2A}$ receptor activity may distinguish ED subgroups after recovery. Furthermore, these data raise the provocative possibility that increased activity of the 5-HT$_{1A}$ receptor may only be found in individuals with bulimic-type symptoms.

Clinical implications

There is a growing understanding of how genetic and neurobiologically mediated mechanisms contribute to a susceptibility to develop EDs. For example, studies of twins with AN and BN support the hypothesis that a significant genetic contribution to liability for AN and BN is accounted for by additive genetic factors (Klump *et al.* 2001). These heritability estimates are in line with those found in studies of schizophrenia and bipolar disorder, suggesting that EDs may be as 'genetically influenced' as disorders traditionally viewed as biological in nature.

Many individuals with AN and BN respond poorly to treatment and/or have a chronic course. In addition, insurance companies are often reluctant to provide adequate treatment, in part because EDs are considered psychosocial in nature or because there is little in the way of evidence-based treatment studies proving the efficacy of therapy. Thus new understandings of the pathogenesis of AN and BN are important for providing a rationale for support for more effective therapy.

The imaging studies done to date show strong and often replicated evidence of powerful disturbances of brain function. Importantly, these findings are present when individuals are ill and persist after recovery. The question can be raised as to whether findings in recovered individuals are 'scars' that are caused by chronic malnutrition or other state-related factors. This is possible, and such questions cannot be fully answered by cross-sectional studies. However, imaging studies in recovered individuals show relationships of alterations to behaviors, such as anxiety, that are now known to occur prior to the onset of AN and BN. This is strong evidence that such brain findings may be traits that are present before the onset of an ED and persist after remission of the diagnosis of AN and BN.

The study of EDs may be at a stage resembling that at which the study of schizophrenia and autism was 20 years ago, when these disorders were also considered psychosocial in nature. It is now well recognized that alterations of brain chemistry contribute to the pathogenesis of schizophrenia and autism. Such data have led to the destigmatization of these illnesses, which in turn has generated support from families, the government, and third-party providers for better treatment and research funding. Moreover, an understanding of how brain pathways may contribute to disorders such as schizophrenia offers the promise of new and better treatments in that illness. Thus it is important that the ED field welcome and utilize these new understandings of the pathophysiology of ED.

Future directions

The limits of technology have led to gross oversimplification in understanding how the brain works. That is, previous studies have used peripheral measures such as hormone levels as an index of 5-HT activity, which was often characterized as low or high. To some extent, imaging studies still suffer from oversimplification in attempting to relate one receptor or one brain region to complex behaviors. It is important to recognize that neuronal activity is an integration of many factors such as neuronal firing, synaptic release and re-uptake, intracellular mechanisms, and interactions with other neuronal systems. The neuronal activity of hundreds of thousands of neurons make up brain circuits. It is likely that in order to understand behavior, we will need to understand the pathophysiology of brain circuits in humans. Individuals with EDs tend to have comorbid depression, anxiety, obsessionality and other symptoms. In the past decade imaging studies have made great advances in understanding brain circuits that contribute to mood and impulse control. Disorders that we consider 'different' by DSM-IV standards, such as depression, OCD, ED, or substance abuse, may in fact each involve many of the same brain regions that modulate mood and impulse control. However, the pattern of disturbances within these pathways may be different for depression versus OCD, etc. The ED field has lagged behind other major psychiatric disorders in terms of understanding brain pathways or developing animal models. However, perhaps more is known about regulation of appetite behavior than is known about mood or impulse control. Thus investigations that seek to understand appetite in AN and BN are likely to result in rapid progress in understanding how the brain functions in people with AN and BN. Finally, brain imaging and genetics hold the promise of being able to characterize complex systems in living humans, and their relationship to behavior. In fact, these tools have rapidly advanced knowledge to the point where we can begin to make educated guesses about the pathophysiology of AN and BN and start to model mechanisms that may be used to test hypotheses.

Acknowledgment

These imaging studies were made possible by the talent and hard work of Claire McConaha, Shannan E Henry, Julie C Price, Carolyn C Meltzer, Scott K Ziolko, Lisa Weissfeld, Chester A Mathis, Jessica Hoge, Kathy Plotnicov, and Eva Gerardi.

Corresponding author: Walter H Kaye, University of Pittsburgh, School of Medicine, Department of Psychiatry, Western Psychiatric Institute and Clinic, Pittsburgh, Pennsylvania, USA. Email: kayewh@upmc.edu

References

References preceded by three asterisks are of particular significance. The significance is explained by a short commentary following the complete reference.

Arana F, Parkinson JA, Hinton E, Holland A, Owen A and Roberts A (2003) Dissociable contributions of the human amygdala and orbitofrontal cortex to incentive motivation and goal selection. *European Journal of Neuroscience*, **23(29)**: 9632–838.
Artmann H, Grau H, Adelmann M and Schleiffer R (1985) Reversible and non-reversible enlargement of cerebrospinal fluid spaces in anorexia nervosa. *Neuroradiology*, **27(4)**: 304–12.

Audenaert K, Van Laere K, Dumont F, Vervaet M, Goethals I, Slegers G, Mertens J, van Heeringen C and Dierckx R (2003) Decreased 5-HT2a receptor binding in patients with anorexia nervosa. *J Nucl Med*, **44(2)**: 163–9.

Bailer UF, Frank GK, Henry SE *et al.* (2005) Altered brain serotonin 5-HT$_{1A}$ receptor binding after recovery from anorexia nervosa measured by positron emission tomography and [^{11}C]WAY100635. *Arch Gen Psychiatry*, **62**: 1032–41.

***Bailer UF, Price JC, Meltzer CC, Mathis CA, Frank GK, Weissfeld L, McConaha CW, Henry SE, Brooks-Achenbach S, Barbarich NC and Kaye WH (2004b) Altered 5-HT$_{2A}$ receptor binding after recovery from bulimia-type anorexia nervosa: relationships to harm avoidance and drive for thinness. *Neuropsychopharmacology*, **29(6)**: 1143–55.

This PET study, which is the first, found that brain serotonin 2A (5-HT$_{2A}$) receptor in women recovered from bulimia-type AN was significantly reduced in the left subgenual cingulate, the left parietal cortex, and the right occipital cortex and also found that activity of this receptor was positively related to harm avoidance and negatively related to novelty seeking in cingulate and temporal regions. This study extends research suggesting that altered 5-HT neuronal system activity persists after recovery from bulimia-type AN, particularly in subgenual cingulate regions, and supports the possibility that this may be a trait-related disturbance that contributes to the pathophysiology of eating disorders.

Barnes NM and Sharp T (1999) A review of central 5-HT receptors and their function. *Neuropharmacology*, **38(8)**: 1083–152.

Cannon C and Bseikri M (2004) Is dopamine required for natural reward? *Physiol Behav*, **81(5)**: 741–8.

Cerf-Ducastel B and Murphy C (2004) Validation of a stimulation protocol suited to the investigation of odor-taste interactions with fMRI. *Physiol Behav*, **81(3)**: 389–96.

***De Araujo I, Rolls E, Kringelbach M, McGlone F and Phillips N (2003) Taste-olfactory convergence, and the representation of the pleasantness of flavour, in the human brain. *Eur Journal of Neuroscience*, **18**: 2059–68.

This article describes human brain regions that are activated by both taste and smell and which include parts of the caudal orbitofrontal cortex, amygdala, insula cortex, and adjoining areas, and anterior cingulate cortex. Recent imaging studies in anorexia and bulimia nervosa suggest that the function of some of these higher-order association cortical areas, which support flavor processing, are altered in eating disorders.

Del Parigi A, Chen K, Gautier J, Salbe A, Pratley R, Ravussin E and Tataranni P (2002) Sex differences in the human brain's response to hunger and satiation. *Am J Clin Nutr*, **75(6)**: 1017–22.

Dolan RJ, Mitchell J and Wakeling A (1988) Structural brain changes in patients with anorexia nervosa. *Psychological Medicine*, **18**: 349–53.

Drewnowski A, Bellisle F, Aimez P and Remy B (1987a) Taste and bulimia. *Physiol Behav*, **41**: 621–6.

Drewnowski A, Halmi KA, Pierce B, Gibbs J and Smith GP (1987b) Taste and eating disorders. *Am J Clin Nutr*, **46(3)**: 442–50.

Ellison Z, Foong J, Howard R, Bullmore E, Williams S and Treasure J (1998) Functional anatomy of calorie fear in anorexia nervosa. *The Lancet*, **352(9135)**: 1192.

Frank G, Meltzer CC, Price J, Drevets WC, Greer P, Mathis C and Kaye WH (2002a) *Alterations of 5-HT1A and 2A Receptors Persist After Recovery from Anorexia and Bulimia Nervosa*. Society of Biological Psychiatry, Philadelphia.

***Frank G, Kaye WH, Meltzer CC, Price JC, Greer P, McConaha C and Skovira K (2002b) Reduced 5-HT2A receptor binding after recovery from anorexia nervosa. *Biol Psychiatry*, **52**: 896–906.

This study showed for the first time in vivo in anorexic women reduced serotonin receptor binding after recovery. Those receptor alterations were found both on a region of interest-based analysis as well as using a whole brain statistical method, in the mesial temporal cortex including the amygdala. This study suggested serotonergic limbic system alterations in an

Frank G, Kaye W, Carter C, Brooks S, May C, Fissel K and Stenger V (2003) The evaluation of brain activity in response to taste stimuli–a pilot study and method for central taste activation as assessed by event related fMRI. *Journal of Neuroscience Methods*, **131(1–2)**: 99–105.

Gagel O (1953) *Magersucht*. Springer, Berlin.

Goethals I, Vervaet M, Audenaert K, Van de Wiele C, Ham H, Vandecapelle M, Slegers G, Dierckx RA and van Heeringen C (2004) Comparison of cortical 5-HT2A receptor binding in bulimia nervosa patients and healthy volunteers. *Am J Psychiatry*, **161(10)**: 1916–18.

Golden NH, Ashtari M, Kohn MR, Patel M, Jacobson MS, Fletcher A and Shenker IR (1996) Reversibility of cerebral ventricular enlargement in anorexia nervosa, demonstrated by quantitative magnetic resonance imaging. *Journal of Pediatrics*, **128**: 296–301.

Gordon CM, Dougherty DD, Fischman AJ, Emans SJ, Grace E, Lamm R, Alpert NM, Majzoub JA and Rausch SL (2001) Neural substrates of anorexia nervosa: a behavioral challenge study with positron emission tomography. *J Pediatr*, **139(1)**: 51–7.

Gottfried JA, O'Doherty J and Dolan RJ (2002) Appetite and aversive olfactory learning in humans studied using event-related functional magnetic resonance imaging. *J Neuroscience*, **15(22)**: 10829–37.

Heinz ER, Martinez J and Haenggeli A (1977) Reversibility of cerebral atrophy in anorexia nervosa and Cushing's syndrome. *Journal of Computer Assisted Tomography*, **1(4)**: 415–18.

Hoffman GW, Ellinwood EHJ, Rockwell WJ, Herfkens RJ, Nishita JK and Guthrie LF (1989) Cerebral atrophy in bulimia. *Biol Psychiatry*, **25**: 894–902.

Husain MM, Black KJ, Doraiswamy PM *et al.* (1992) Subcortical brain anatomy in anorexia and bulimia. *Biol Psychiatry*, **31**: 735–8.

Katzman DK, Lambe EK, Mikulis DJ, Ridgley JN, Goldbloom DS and Zipursky RB (1996) Cerebral gray matter and white matter volume deficits in adolescent girls with anorexia nervosa. *Journal of Pediatrics*, **129**: 794–803.

Katzman DK, Zipursky RB, Lambe EK and Mikulis DJ (1997) A longitudinal magnetic resonance imaging study of brain changes in adolescents with anorexia nervosa. *Arch Pediatr Adolesc Med*, **151(8)**: 793–7.

Kaye WH, Frank GK, Meltzer CC, Price JC, McConaha CW, Crossan PJ, Klump KL and Rhodes L (2001) Altered serotonin 2A receptor activity in women who have recovered from bulimia nervosa. *Am J Psychiatry*, **158(7)**: 1152–5.

Kaye W, Frank G, Bailer U, Wagner A, Henry S, McConaha C, Vogel V, Meltzer C, Price J and Mathis C (2004) *Defining the Neuroanatomy of Anorexia and Bulimia Nervosa*. Eating Disorders Research Society, Amsterdam, The Netherlands.

Killgore W, Young A, Femia L, Bogorodzki P, Rogowska J and Yurgelun-Todd D (2003) Cortical and limbic activation during viewing of high- versus low-calorie foods. *Neuroimage*, **19(4)**: 1381–94.

Kingston K, Szmukler G, Andrewes D, Tress B and Desmond P (1996) Neuropsychological and structural brain changes in anorexia nervosa before and after refeeding. *Psychol Med*, **26(1)**: 15–28.

Klump KL, Kaye WH and Strober M (2001) The evolving genetic foundations of eating disorders. *Psychiatr Clin North Am*, **24(2)**: 215–25.

Kohlmeyer K, Lehmkuhl G and Poustka F (1983) Computed tomography of anorexia nervosa. *AJNR*, **4**: 437–8.

Krieg JC, Pirke KM, Lauer C and Backmund H (1988) Endocrine, metabolic, and cranial computed tomographic findings in AN. *Biol Psychiatry*, **23**: 377–87.

Krieg JC, Lauer C and Pirke KM (1989) Structural brain abnormalities in patients with bulimia nervosa. *Psychiatry Research*, **27**: 39–48.

Kringelbach ML, de Araujo IET and Rolls ET (2004) Taste-related activity in the human dorsolateral prefrontal cortex. *Neuro-image*, **21**: 781–8.

Kronreich L, Shapira A, Horev G, Danzinger Y, Tyano S and Moimouni M (1991) CT and MR evaluation of the brain in patients with anorexia nervosa. *American Journal of Neuroradiology*, **12**: 1213–16.

LaBar K, Gitelman D, Parrish T, Kim Y, Nobre A and Mesulam M (2001) Hunger selectively modulates corticolimbic activation to food stimuli in humans. *Behav Neurosci*, **115(2)**: 493–500.

Laessle RG, Krieg JC, Fichter MM and Pirke KM (1989) Cerebral atrophy and vigilance performance in patients with anorexia and bulimia nervosa. *Neuropsychobiology*, **21(4)**: 187–91.

Lambe EK, Katzman DK, Mikulis DJ, Kennedy SH and Zipursky RB (1997) Cerebral gray matter volume deficits after weight recovery from anorexia nervosa. *Arch Gen Psychiatry*, **54(6)**: 537–42.

Lankenau H, Swigar M, Bhimani S, Luchins D and Quainlan D (1985) Cranial CT scans in eating disorder patients and controls. *Compr Psychiatry*, **26(2)**: 136–47.

Martin F (1958) Patholoie des aspects neurologiques et psychiatriques des quelques manifestations carentielles avec troubles digestifs et neuro-endocriniens: etude des alterations du systeme nerveux central dans deux cas d'anorexie survenue chez la jeune fille (dite anorexie mentale). *Acta Neurologica Belgica*, **52**: 816–30.

McClure S, Li J, Tomlin D, Cypert K, Montague L and Montague P (2004) Neural correlates of behavioral preference for culturally familiar drinks. *Neuron*, **44(2)**: 379–87.

Naruo T, Nakabeppu Y, Sagiyama K, Munemoto T, Homan N, Deguchi D, Nakajo M and Nozoe S (2000) Characteristic regional cerebral blood flow patterns in anorexia nervosa patients with binge/purge behavior. *Am J Psychiatry*, **157(9)**: 1520–2.

Neumarker KJ, Bzufka WM, Dudeck U, Hein J and Neumarker U (2000) Are there specific disabilities of number processing in adolescent patients with anorexia nervosa? Evidence from clinical and neuropsychological data when compared to morphometric measures from magnetic resonance imaging. *European Child and Adolescent Psychiatry*, **9**: 111–21.

Nozoe S, Naruo T, Nakabeppu Y, Soejima Y, Nakajo M and Tanaka H (1993) Changes in regional cerebral blood flow in patients with anorexia nervosa detected through single photon emission tomography imaging. *Biol Psychiatry*, **34(8)**: 578–80.

Nozoe S, Naruo T, Yonekura R, Nakabeppu Y, Soejima Y, Nagai N, Nakajo M and Tanaka H (1995) Comparison of regional cerebral blood flow in patients with eating disorders. *Brain Res Bull*, **36(3)**: 251–5.

Nussbaum M, Shenker IR, Marc J and Klein M (1980) Cerebral atrophy in anorexia nervosa. *Journal of Pediatrics*, **96(5)**: 867–9.

Palazidou E, Robinson PS and Lishman WA (1990) Neuroradiological and neuropsychological assessment in anorexia nervosa. *Psychol Med*, **20(3)**: 521–7.

Schoenfeld M, Neuer G, Tempelmann C, Schussler K, Noesselt T, Hopf J and Heinze H (2004) Functional magnetic resonance tomography correlates of taste perception in the human primary taste cortex. *Neuroscience*, **127(2)**: 347–53.

Seeger G, Braus DF, Ruf M, Goldberger U and Schmidt MH (2002) Body image distortion reveals amygdala activation in patients with anorexia nervosa – a functional magnetic resonance imaging study. *Neuroscience Letters*, **326**: 25–8.

Shirao N, Okamoto Y, Okada G, Okamoto Y and Yamawaki S (2003) Temporomesial activation in young females associated with unpleasant words concerning body image. *Neuropsychobiology*, **48(3)**: 136–42.

Small D, Jones-Gotman M and Dagher A (2003) Feeding-induced dopamine release in dorsal striatum correlates with meal pleasantness ratings in healthy human volunteers. *Neuro-image*, **19(4)**: 1709–15.

Swayze VW, Andersen A, Arndt S, Rajarethinam R, Fleming F, Sato Y and Andreasen NC (1996) Reversibility of brain tissue loss in anorexia nervosa assessed with a computerized Talairach 3-D proportional grid. *Psychol Med*, **26(2)**: 381–90.

Swayze VW II, Andersen AE, Andreasen NC, Arndt S, Sato Y and Ziebell S (2003) Brain tissue volume segmentation in patients with anorexia nervosa before and after weight normalization. *Int J Eat Disord*, **33(1)**: 33–44.

Takano A, Shiga T, Kitagava N *et al.* (2001) Abnormal neuronal network in anorexia nervosa studied with I-123-IMP SPECT. *Psychiatry Research: Neuroimaging*, **107(1)**: 45–50.

Tauscher J, Pirker W, Willeit M, de Zwaan M, Bailer U, Neumeister A, Asenbaum S, Lennkh N, Praschak-Rieder N, Brücke T and Kasper S (2001) [^{123}I]beta-CIT and single photon emission computed tomography reveal reduced brain serotonin transporter availability in bulimia nervosa. *Biol Psychiatry*, **49(4)**: 326–32.

Tiihonen J, Keski-Rahkonen A, Lopponen M, Muhonen M, Kajander J, Allonen T, Nagren K, Hietala J and Rissanen A (2004) Brain serotonin 1A receptor binding in bulimia nervosa. *Biol Psychiatry*, **55**: 871–3.

Uher R, Brammer M, Murphy T, Campbell I, Ng V, Williams S and Treasure J (2003) Recovery and chronicity in anorexia nervosa: brain activity associated with differential outcomes. *Biological Psychiatry*, **54**: 934–42.

***Uher R, Murphy T, Brammer M, Dalgleish T, Phillips M, Ng V, Andrew C, Williams S, Campbell I and Treasure J (2004) Medial prefrontal cortex activity associated with symptom provocation in eating disorders. *Am J Psychiatry*, **161(7)**: 1238–46.

This study, which is the largest to date, used fMRI to understand response to food and other stimuli in women with eating disorders and found greater activation in the left medial orbitofrontal and anterior cingulate cortices and less activation in the lateral prefrontal cortex relative to the comparison group. An abnormal propensity to activate medial prefrontal circuits in response to inappropriate stimuli may be common to eating, obsessive–compulsive, and addictive disorders and may contribute to compulsive features in these conditions.

***Wagner A, Ruf M, Braus DF and Schmidt MH (2003) Neuronal activity changes and body image distortion in anorexia nervosa. *NeuroReport*, **14(17)**: 2193–7.

This is the first functional brain imaging study in a convincing sample size of ill anorectic adolescents assessing body-image distortion by confronting them with digitally distorted images. Parietal lobe activation seems to be associated with this disturbance. The most striking finding is the difference in activation pattern in this brain region in response to their own body image compared to a picture of a different person indicating differences in visuo-spatial processing.

Wagner A, Aizenstein H, Frank G, Figurski J, May C, Fischer L, Bailer U, Henry S, McConaha C, Vogel V and Kaye W (2004) *Neuronal activation in response to taste stimuli – an fMRI study*. Neuropsychopharmacology, ACNP 43rd Annual Meeting, San Juan, Puerto Rico.

Wang G, Volkow ND, Telang F, Jayne M, Ma J, Rao M, Zhu W, Wong C, Pappas N, Geliebter A and Fowler J (2004) Exposure to appetitive food stimuli markedly activates the human brain. *Neuro-image*, **21(4)**: 1790–7.

Zeumer H, Hacke W and Hartwich P (1982) A quantitative approach to measuring the cerebrospinal fluid space with CT. *Neuroradiology*, **22**: 193–7.

8

Eating disorders in children and adolescents

Rachel J Bryant-Waugh

Abstract

Objectives of review. To review papers published in 2003 and 2004 specifically relating to the clinical management of children and adolescents with eating disorders (EDs), and to identify main current areas of interest and research activity.

Summary of recent findings. Although there have been many publications relating to EDs in young patients during 2003–2004, there were no controlled treatment trials. Recent findings include evidence that adolescence remains a period of high risk for both AN and BN, and that outcome in AN remains relatively poor with up to half experiencing persisting psychiatric problems up to 10 years later. Rate of weight gain whilst in hospital is emerging as a factor predictive of outcome for AN. Developments in individual psychological interventions have included motivational approaches and the use of monitored exercise in underweight patients during refeeding. Treatment of choice for pubertal delay and bone complications is still normalization of dietary intake and weight restoration, and the use of medication in general is not recommended as a first-line choice of treatment for the ED. Effective family interventions have been described and evaluated, both for AN and BN.

Future directions. It is recommended that attention is paid to diagnostic and classification issues, and that specific developmentally appropriate interventions for the full range of ED presentations seen in this age group are subjected to proper evaluation. Controlled treatment trials are very much needed, and might help reduce some of the variability in guidelines and recommendations currently available to clinicians working with this age group.

Introduction

The years 2003–2004 have seen the publication of a number of systematic reviews, position papers from professional bodies, and national guidelines relating to EDs. Many of these have separate sections or recommendations regarding specific aspects of the identification, assessment and treatment of EDs in children and adolescents (e.g. NICE 2004; Royal Australian and New Zealand College of Psychiatrists 2004), and some are devoted entirely to this younger age group (e.g. American Academy of Pediatrics 2003; Ebeling *et al.* 2003; Rome *et al.* 2003). Additionally, a number of more general chapters, papers and books have been published during this period that discuss EDs in children and adolescents from a variety of perspectives. Some are intended for clinicians and researchers (e.g. Birmingham and Beumont 2004; Linscheid and Butz 2003; Kreipe and Yussman 2003; Nicholls and Bryant-Waugh 2003; Sigman 2003), and others for parents or carers (e.g. Bryant-Waugh and Lask 2004; Lock and Le Grange 2005). A wide range of research and discussion papers involving or specifically focusing on issues relevant to children and adolescents have also been added to the literature, although randomized controlled treatment trials in this age group have remained conspicuous by their absence during the period covered here.

The aim of this chapter is to draw together some of the main areas of clinical interest and research activity regarding children and adolescents with EDs published in 2003 and 2004, paying particular attention to those with direct clinical relevance or implications in terms of patient care and service development. This chapter is not a comprehensive or systematic review, but one that hopefully captures current activity and interest, and recent developments relevant to treating young people with EDs, whilst pointing the interested reader in the direction of further detail. Please note that since many chapters in Part 1 of the AED Annual Report series, as well as in this volume, contain sections relevant to children and adolescents, attempts have been made to avoid unnecessary duplication. Useful material relating to children and adolescents can additionally be found elsewhere (*see further* Wonderlich *et al.* 2005).

Literature review

Update on classification and diagnostic issues

The classification of eating disturbances in childhood remains a subject of much discussion (Rosen 2003) with many within the field calling for more flexible, developmentally appropriate criteria. It seems fairly clear that current diagnostic systems are rather limited in their scope and do not satisfactorily capture the full range of clinically significant presentations, where disturbance of eating is a main feature, seen in the younger age group. Some such presentations are likely to fall within the existing EDNOS category, that is, very closely related to AN and BN. Others might more appropriately fall under alternative existing categories (e.g. childhood presentations of other existing psychiatric disturbances and disorders such as anxiety or somatoform disorders), or even belong in as-yet-undefined categories of their own (for example, as specific variants of developmental disorder or childhood-onset behavioral and emotional disorder). The diagnostic debate in relation to childhood presentations of psychiatric disorders is not unique to EDs, and the ongoing confusion undoubtedly presents problems in terms of developing and disseminating effective treatment interventions for this age group, as well as of attempting to gain a reliable picture of clinical need. A number of authors have made suggestions for improvement: Marcus and Kalarchian (2003) propose developmentally appropriate provisional BED research criteria for children, whilst Chatoor and Surles (2004) propose new diagnostic criteria for 'infantile anorexia', 'sensory food aversions' and 'post-traumatic ED' to fill the gap between feeding disorders and early-onset AN and BN. Other authors continue to use a range of other descriptive terms, e.g. 'selective eating', 'food avoidance emotional disorder' (e.g. Nicholls and Bryant-Waugh 2003). Whilst such terms undoubtedly have good face validity, and represent a useful means of prompting further work in this area, other important aspects of deriving diagnostic systems in relation to childhood eating disturbances have been largely ignored (*see* section on Future directions, p.138).

Incidence and prevalence of EDs in children and adolescents

The epidemiology of EDs is reviewed in Chapter 4 by Striegel-Moore. Whereas incidence rates for full syndrome AN (where adolescents form the population at highest risk) do not seem to be increasing significantly (Milos *et al.* 2004), emerging evidence from one UK study suggests that the risk for BN may now be highest in 10–19 year olds, due to incidence rates in adult women dropping off in recent years (Currin *et al.* 2005). As age ranges studied and diagnostic criteria employed vary considerably in epidemiological studies, it is extremely difficult to get a clear picture of incidence and prevalence rates of EDs and atypical EDs for children and adolescents as separate groups.

One important purpose of epidemiological studies is to inform appropriate service development and to promote adequate healthcare provision. Another way to assess the level of need for clinical services is to audit current service use. A recent study reported the results of a one-day census of the diagnoses of resident patients in 71 inpatient units in England and Wales treating children and adolescents with a mental illness (O'Herlihy *et al.* 2004): 23% of all patients over 13 and 15% of those under 13 had a diagnosis of ED on the day of the census. In the over-13s this represented the largest diagnostic group, and in the under-13s, the second largest group. Young people with EDs were found to occupy more child and adolescent mental health beds than young people with any other diagnosis.

Service and general treatment issues

There remains significant variation in recommended treatment approaches for young people with EDs, with some guidelines and authors emphasizing medical monitoring and related interventions much more strongly than others. Most young patients with AN, BN and related EDs are managed on an outpatient basis, with inpatient care being recommended for a minority with AN, where there are serious complications related to comorbid diagnoses, or where there is high physical and/or psychiatric risk (Nicholls and Bryant-Waugh 2003). The NICE guidelines recommend that a number of factors, including social and educational needs, should be taken into account when considering whether to admit a young person. Usually, such a decision tends to rest heavily on medical concerns. For example, the American Academy of Pediatrics recommends admission on the basis of the following features: less than 75% weight for height, or ongoing weight loss; refusal to eat; body fat level less than 10%; pulse under 50 by day and under 45 by night; systolic pressure < 90; presence of orthostatic changes in pulse or blood pressure; body temperature < 96° F; presence of cardiac arrhythmia (American Academy of Pediatrics 2003). However, not all clinicians believe that it is necessary to admit even very underweight children to hospital, although this must in most cases depend on the availability of good outpatient services and motivated, supportive family members.

Most guidelines emphasize the need for a comprehensive approach to treatment, involving multidisciplinary team input, with medical and psychological as well as social and educational aspects of treatment. The importance of separate input for parents and carers has also been recognized, with focus groups and service user/carer initiatives clearly identifying needs for support, involvement and education of family members (NICE 2004).

Other aspects of the clinical management of EDs, in particular AN, which have acquired greater prominence in recent years are those related to the young person's capacity to make decisions and to consent to treatment (e.g. Tan et al. 2003). The difficulties of engaging young people who may not view themselves as ill (and usually do not wish to gain weight), maintaining a therapeutic alliance with an ambivalent or 'resistant' patient, and the ethical dilemmas posed when health deteriorates still further, at times necessitating feeding against the will of the patient, present a considerable challenge to clinicians (NICE 2004).

Weight restoration in AN and other low-weight presentations

Clinical practice and protocols still vary in terms of how weight gain can best be achieved in underweight patients, and the level of medical monitoring that goes with this process–some clinicians are reluctant to submit children with AN to multiple medical tests and investigations, whilst others would strongly regard this as an important aspect of responsible and appropriate physical care. Rome and colleagues suggest that adolescents treated as inpatients can be expected to achieve a weight gain of 0.9–1.25 kg per week, whilst those managed on an outpatient basis can be expected to gain 0.45–0.9 kg per week (Rome et al. 2003). NICE (2004) suggests 0.5–1 kg per week for inpatients, and up to 0.5 kg for outpatients.

In young people who have had minimal dietary intake for some time, care needs to be taken to avoid 'refeeding syndrome' (a term covering a range of potentially lethal electrolyte and biochemical disturbances that may result from a sudden increase in metabolic load accompanying a rapid rise in dietary intake). A paced approach to increasing energy intake is recommended in such young people, combined with some level of physical monitoring (*see* Ebeling *et al.* 2003; Golden and Meyer 2004 for recommendations specific to adolescents).

Management of medical complications and other physical aspects

An episode of AN during late childhood/early adolescence interferes with the normal growth and development processes of puberty and of accruing peak bone density, in turn related to the development of osteopenia and osteoporosis. The main recommended treatment for pubertal delay and bone complications in younger patients remains weight restoration and normalization of dietary intake (with the aim of prompting spontaneous progress through puberty with onset or resumption of menses), with vitamin D and calcium supplementation as required. Heer *et al.* (2004) report improved concentrations of bone formation markers in 19 adolescent patients with AN following nutritional therapy. Trials involving biphosphonates, dehydroepiandrosterone (DHEA), and insulin-like growth factor (IGF-I) have shown some promise, but these preparations are not currently considered the mainstay of treatment for bone density problems in adolescents (Golden 2003). Wentz and colleagues found that bone mineral density (BMD) was similar in a group of young adult females an average of 11 years after teenage-onset AN compared to a healthy female comparison group. These authors comment, however, that the three males in the group had lower BMD than control males, and also that they found an inverse relationship between BMD and AN duration, which may indicate risk for osteopenia in those only partially recovered or those with chronic AN (Wentz *et al.* 2003). The use of estrogen preparations to address bone density concerns is not recommended in children and adolescents because of the risk of premature fusion of epiphyses and compromised adult height (NICE 2004). Weight levels at which menstruation returns in adolescents who have established regular menses prior to the onset of their AN are highly variable, and Swenne (2004) suggests on the basis of his investigations that population-based target weights such as those usually set may be too generalized or too low, recommending instead that where possible targets should be individually set, based on premorbid trajectories and values.

Pharmacological treatment

Recommendations on the use of medication in the treatment of adolescents with EDs are reviewed and summarized in Gowers and Bryant-Waugh (2004): no form of medication currently forms a first-line choice of treatment for AN, but appropriate drugs may be used in the treatment of comorbid diagnoses and symptoms, especially anxiety. Fluoxetine may be prescribed in weight-restored adolescents with AN, with supplementary multivitamins, calcium, zinc, iron and folate used as required (Rome *et al.* 2003). The dangers of prescribing drugs with cardiac side-effects to severely malnourished patients who may have electrolyte disturbances, and who are at risk of cardiac complications have been emphasized (NICE 2004), with some authors concluding that the use of such medication should be reserved for young people whose weight has been restored (Ebeling *et al.* 2003). Case reports that the use of olanzapine in children with AN has been well tolerated and associated with considerable clinical improvement have led to calls for further studies to determine safety and effectiveness in this age group (Boachie *et al.* 2003). Additionally, Rome and colleagues suggest that where delayed gastric emptying is impeding refeeding, metoclopramide can be prescribed (Rome *et al.* 2003). This group further suggests that where purging or reflux has resulted in esophagitis, histamine-2 blockers and/or proton-pump inhibitors can be used (Rome *et al.* 2003). Finally, Ebeling and colleagues suggest that short-acting benzodiazepines can be administered before meals to decrease anxiety (Ebeling *et al.* 2003).

On the basis of their review of the drug studies in BN, Ebeling and colleagues simply conclude that 'there is no evidence justifying the use of medication as the only or primary treatment for bulimia in children and adolescents' (Ebeling *et al.* 2003). NICE similarly concludes that there is no evidence supporting the practice of using antidepressants in the treatment of adolescent BN, and that they should not be considered as a first-line treatment (NICE 2004).

Psychological therapies

Family interventions

In recent years a move towards a widespread acceptance of the importance of family interventions in the treatment of children and adolescents with EDs has been seen. The NICE guidelines stress that some family-based psychological intervention, normally to include siblings, should form part of the treatment of EDs in this age group. Optimal 'family interventions that directly address the ED', recommended for AN (NICE 2004, p. 90), require further exploration, development, and evaluation, but will usually involve information sharing, a focus on behavioral management and facilitation of communication between family members. In the past few years there have been a number of papers describing such interventions and providing further evidence of potential for effectiveness, thereby encouraging work in this area. For example, Krautter and Lock (2004) and Le Grange *et al.* (2005) describe the use of a manualized family-based treatment for AN, and Eisler *et al.* (2003) summarize developments in the use of multiple family therapy in the treatment of adolescent EDs. Family relationships of adolescent patients with AN continue to be studied, with pointers emerging for specific issues to be considered and addressed as appropriate in family interventions. For example, Karwautz and colleagues found that adolescent girls with AN had lower perceived individual autonomy than their well sisters, and that this difference was largely attributable to their relationship with their mothers, and to a lesser extent with their fathers (Karwautz *et al.* 2003). Alongside these developments, others have applied progress in other areas of psychological theory and therapy to family-based treatment of young people with EDs. For example, Dallos (2003) utilizes developments in attachment theory and narrative approaches in family interventions in the management of EDs.

Other authors have continued to develop family-based interventions for adolescents with BN: for example, Le Grange *et al.* (2003) provide a useful description of one such development that is currently being further investigated in a randomized controlled trial. Support for family interventions in bulimic adolescents comes additionally from studies such as that by Okon *et al.* (2003) who investigated triggers of binge eating in 20 adolescent girls (mean age 16.8) with BN. They found that family interaction has a significant impact on symptom variation, with family hassles predicting bulimic episodes in those adolescents who perceived their family as characterized by high conflict or low emotional expressiveness.

Individual interventions

There is still some way to go in the development and evaluation of individual therapies for young people with EDs, with a need for specifically tailored treatments suitable for different types of presentation, which are developmentally appropriate. Decaluwe *et al.* (2003) highlight the need for obese children with binge-eating problems to have tailored interventions, given their finding of a tendency towards lower self-esteem and higher levels of eating, weight and shape concerns in binge-eating obese children compared to nonbinge-eating obese children. Isnard and colleagues also found that obese adolescents engaging in binge eating had higher levels of psychological distress, particularly on dimensions of anxiety, signaling the need for adapted interventions (Isnard *et al.* 2003).

With regard to AN, alongside family interventions, some individual work will usually be required. The use of motivational approaches, well described with adults, has begun to be explored with adolescents presenting for treatment of AN. Gowers and Smyth (2004) investigated whether the addition of a motivational interview at assessment changed self-reported motivation in 42 adolescents with AN, and whether it had a positive influence on engagement with treatment and early behavioral change. They demonstrated a significant positive effect on motivation scores, with motivational status predicting engagement and weight gain, encouraging them to proceed to planning a randomized controlled trial. Other individual interventions can be informed by studies such as that by Holtkamp *et al.* (2004), who investigated the relationships between dietary restriction, physical activity and psychopathology in 30 adolescents admitted for treatment of AN. They concluded that anxiety symptoms and dietary restriction may synergistically contribute to increased levels of exercise, and in their discussion of the clinical implications of their findings, caution that restriction of physical activity during refeeding may further increase anxiety and stress, which in turn can create problems for full engagement in treatment efforts. A detailed account of one approach to actively incorporating physical exercise in the treatment of AN is given by Duesund and Skårderud (2003), in their exploration of how engagement in activity can shift the focus away from the anorexic negative experience of the body. In terms of working with body-image disturbance issues, Gusella *et al.* (2004) report the findings of a study involving 22 girls diagnosed with EDs, all of whom had a negative view of their body appearance, but a relatively positive view in terms of body function. These authors suggest that making a distinction between body appearance and function might prove clinically useful in addressing body-image disturbance.

No controlled treatment trials of adolescents with BN were published in the period included in this review, although these are imminent. NICE (2004) concludes that subject to adaptation for age and level of development, adolescents with BN may be treated in a similar way to adults with the disorder (i.e. based on a specific form of cognitive behavior therapy–CBT-BN), though consideration should be given to involvement of the family. The use of cognitive therapy in the treatment of adolescent EDs more generally is described by Bowers *et al.* (2003).

Group interventions

Again, group interventions for children and adolescents with EDs need to be developmentally appropriate, and require further development and evaluation before specific recommendations can be made. Given the importance of peer relationships during adolescence, and the impact of social functioning on treatment, developments such as a group intervention focussing on friendship issues in hospitalized anorexic adolescents, described by Davies (2004), are of interest.

Outcome

Outcome and follow-up studies of young people with EDs inevitably vary in terms of their findings. This is likely to be in part related to problems around lack of comparability between subjects (due to unresolved diagnostic issues discussed above) and in part, due to differences in terms of treatment received. A recent study from Norway found that of 51 patients with child- and adolescent-onset AN treated 3.5 to 14.5 years previously, 82% had no ED at follow-up, but 41% had one or more other axis-I psychiatric diagnosis, with depression and anxiety disorders being the most common (Halvorsen *et al.* 2004). The picture of a reasonably good overall outcome for most patients in terms of ED symptoms, but ongoing mental health problems in a significant number, seems fairly consistent. Råstam *et al.* (2003) found that in their 10-year follow-up of a similar number of adolescent-onset AN patients, around half were free from their ED, but around one-quarter persisted in having an ED, mostly AN. These authors found that affective disorders tended to resolve with the ED, but that obsessive–compulsive and autistic spectrum disturbances persisted in more than one-third of the AN cases, with half the original group having an overall poor outcome. Fisher (2003) concludes that the outcome literature seems to suggest that overall, adolescents with EDs do somewhat better than adults, but that it is not clear how large this difference is.

A number of authors have further investigated or reported on predictors of outcome in younger patients. Rome and colleagues conclude that in young patients with AN, those with purging subtype tend to do better than those with restricting subtype, the opposite to that reported in many adult studies (Rome *et al.* 2003). The same investigators observed that premorbid asociality and exercise compulsion (common in young patients with AN) predicted poor outcome. In another study, designed to determine which variables at first admission are related to the need for readmission, Castro *et al.* (2004) found that 24.8% of 101 11–19 year olds treated for AN required readmission after complete weight recovery, with lower rate of weight gain, lower mean age and more abnormal eating, weight, and shape attitudes most clearly related to rehospitalization. Lock and Litt (2003) reported that response to initial hospitalization (in terms of weight gain) predicted better outcomes at 12 months in 41 adolescent patients, rather than admission weight or length of stay. A study from Italy, investigating natural outcome in 12 adolescents identified in a screening study as having full, partial syndrome and subclinical EDs, found that four years later none had received treatment and that seven of the eight subclinical cases had remitted, but the full and partial syndrome cases had remained stable (Cotrufo *et al.* 2004).

Summary of important findings and areas of interest

The years 2003 and 2004 have seen the publication of different sets of recommendations and guidelines pertaining to the management and treatment of children and adolescents with EDs, most acknowledging the importance of multidisciplinary input combining medical, psychological, social and educational components, and the involvement of the family. There remains considerable variation in the detail of these recommendations, probably related to the method by which they were derived and the emphasis placed on different sources of knowledge (i.e. systematic reviews of available research evidence, expert consensus, etc.). Classification and diagnostic issues have received more attention recently, with an increase in awareness around the problems related to the current available systems. It remains difficult to be precise about exact numbers of young people who have EDs, but recent reports make it clear that adolescence represents a period of major risk for both AN and BN, and related disorders. It has also been shown that amongst all young people requiring admission for treatment of any psychiatric disorder, those with EDs represent one of the largest groups. The role of pharmacological treatments in the management of EDs in children and adolescents remains under-researched and controversial. They are generally not recommended in this age group as first-line choices, although appropriate use of medication for comorbid psychiatric symptoms may be helpful. Attention has been drawn to specific constellations of factors that can act as maintaining factors, and attempts made at means of addressing these (e.g. including physical activity alongside refeeding, focusing on developmentally appropriate peer relationship issues, etc.). Finally, we have seen that despite developments in clinical practice, outcome of AN in particular remains relatively poor, with around half of all patients presenting with continuing psychiatric problems at follow-up.

Clinical implications

One important clinical implication to emerge from the above is the reinforcement of the recommendation that in young underweight patients, weight restoration to a level sufficient to restore normal development and to promote spontaneous progress through puberty, with onset or resumption of menses, is paramount. In practice, this means that clinicians treating young patients who are not gaining weight satisfactorily are required to urgently consider alternatives or additional interventions. A further implication relates to the need for specialist education and training on EDs for all child and adolescent practitioners, and willingness for clinicians to actively involve parents, carers and other family members in treatment. Recent research has also supported the notion that some features that can be very difficult to treat and overcome, such as the excessive exercising commonly seen in adolescent AN, might be better managed in more active ways. In this example, a graded, monitored exercise program might be more effective than bedrest.

Future directions

Alongside calls for a revision of existing classification schemes for EDs more generally (e.g. Fairburn and Harrison 2003; Hebebrand *et al.* 2004), the need for this seems particularly acute with regard to this younger population. It seems essential at this stage that proper attention is paid to pertinent elements of both diagnostic validity and clinical utility in relation to any future proposals around classifying childhood eating disturbances, and that due consideration is given to recommendations around revising diagnostic criteria and proposed strategies for evaluating the validity of clinical syndromes (e.g. Kendall and Jablensky 2003; First *et al.* 2004). There is a very long way to go in this regard, and the studies necessary to achieve considerable progress in this respect regrettably appear relatively low down on research priority agendas.

In addition to being able to better define and describe the full range of ED presentations in children and adolescents, there is a need to continue to develop and evaluate tailored, developmentally appropriate interventions. In 2002 the National Institutes of Health convened a workshop on overcoming barriers to treatment research in AN. Its recommendations include the need to improve early recognition of AN in adolescents, to facilitate early treatment when outcomes are most likely to be favorable, and to encourage large-scale psychological intervention studies, which includes supporting innovative treatment approaches and pilot research efforts that can guide such large-scale studies (Agras *et al*. 2004). Further research is required around developing and applying age-appropriate modifications of evidence-based treatments for adult BN to the treatment of adolescents, as well as clarification of the benefits, costs and effectiveness across a range of parameters including physical, psychological, and social, of different service models (inpatient, outpatient, day-patient, specialist and generic settings) in the management of young people with the full range of EDs (Gowers and Bryant-Waugh 2004). The current gaps in knowledge about effective treatments in child and adolescent EDs suggest that almost any adequately powered well-conducted trials would be worthwhile. Particular areas of interest include evaluation of psychological therapies, which effectively address underlying cognitive disturbances as well as promote behavioral change, and are designed to be delivered on an outpatient basis (as this is where most young people are treated) to the full range of clinical presentations seen.

Evaluation of interventions to improve motivation and adherence to treatment is particularly required in this younger population, as many children and adolescents are brought to treatment by others rather than actively seeking treatment themselves, as well as further studies to investigate the relative merits of individual, family or combination treatments. Patient and parent perspectives on treatment experience and satisfaction should be sought in an attempt to contribute towards improved service delivery. Further clarification is needed about subgroups within 'atypical' or 'not otherwise specified' EDs in childhood. Given that there are no evidence-based treatments for this latter heterogeneous group, much work remains to be done to clarify whether treatments for AN and BN may be effective and acceptable to at least a subset of these patients. Predictors of outcome within this group also need further study, as part of a process of improving the ability to match interventions to individual presentations. Finally, we have seen that in clinical practice, there remain considerable differences in how young people with EDs are treated, for example with regard to AN, the recommended extent of accompanying medical intervention and monitoring. Such discrepancies may reflect differences between countries in terms of healthcare delivery systems and insurance issues, but on a more local level, to some extent seem to reflect the nature of the treating team just as much as the disorder being treated. Further investigation into the efficacy of a whole range of components forming part of a comprehensive approach to treatment is certainly required to reduce the extent of variations in treatment recommendations currently available to clinicians.

Corresponding author: Rachel J Bryant-Waugh, Hampshire Partnership NHS Trust Eating Disorder Service, Unit 3 Eastleigh Community Enterprise Centre, Barton Park, Hants SO55 6RR, UK. Email: Rachel.Bryant-waugh@ntlworld.com

References

References preceded by three asterisks are of particular significance. The significance is explained by a short commentary following the complete reference.

Agras S, Brandt H, Bulik C, Dolan-Sewell R, Fairburn C, Halmi K, Herzog D, Jimerson D, Kaplan A, Kaye W, Le Grange D, Lock J, Mitchell J, Rudorfer M, Street L, Striegel-Moore R, Vitousek K, Walsh T and Wilfley D (2004) Report on the National Institutes of Health Workshop on Overcoming Barriers to Treatment Research in Anorexia Nervosa. *International Journal of Eating Disorders*, **35**: 509–21.

American Academy of Pediatrics (2003) Identifying and treating EDs. Policy Statement. *Pediatrics*, **111**: 204–11.

Birmingham L and Beumont P (2004) Prepubertal children and younger adolescents. In: L Birmingham and P Beumont (eds), *Medical Management of Eating Disorders*. Cambridge University Press, Cambridge, pp 184–203.

Boachie A, Goldfield G and Spettigue W (2003) Olanzapine as an adjunctive treatment for hospitalized children with anorexia nervosa: case reports. *International Journal of Eating Disorders*, **33**: 98–103.

Bowers W, Evans K, Le Grange D and Andersen A (2003) Cognitive therapy for adolescent eating disorders. In: M Reinecke, F Dattilio and A Freeman (eds), *Cognitive Therapy for Children and Adolescents: a casebook for clinical practice* (2e). Guilford Press, New York, pp 247–80.

Bryant-Waugh R and Lask B (2004) *Eating Disorders: a parents' guide* (revised edn). Brunner Routledge, Hove, East Sussex.

Castro J, Gila A, Puig J, Rodriguez S and Toro J (2004) Predictors of rehospitalization after total weight recovery in adolescents with AN. *International Journal of Eating Disorders*, **36**: 22–30.

Chatoor I and Surles J (2004) Eating disorders in mid-childhood. *Primary Psychiatry*, **11**: 34–9.

Cotrufo P, Monteleone P, Castaldo E and Maj M (2004) A 4 year epidemiological study of typical and atypical EDs: preliminary evidence for subgroups of atypical EDs with different outcomes. *European Eating Disorders Review*, **12**: 234–9.

Currin L, Schmidt U, Treasure J and Jick H (2005) Time trends in ED incidence. *British Journal of Psychiatry*, **186**: 132–5.

Dallos R (2003) Using narrative and attachment theory in systemic family therapy with EDs. *Clinical Child Psychology and Psychiatry*, **8**: 521–35.

Davies S (2004) A group-work approach to addressing friendship issues in the treatment of adolescents with AN. *Clinical Child Psychology and Psychiatry*, **9**: 519–31.

Decaluwé V, Braet C and Fairburn C (2003) Binge eating in obese children and adolescents. *International Journal of Eating Disorders*, **33**: 78–84.

Duesund L and Skårderud F (2003) Use the body and forget the body: treating AN with Adapted Physical Activity. *Clinical Child Psychology and Psychiatry*, **8**: 53–72.

Ebeling H, Tapanainen P, Joutsenoja A, Koskinen M, Morin-Papunen L, Järvi L, Hassinen R, Keski-Rahkonen A, Rissanen A and Wahlbeck K (2003) Practice guideline for treatment of EDs in children and adolescents. *Annals of Medicine*, **35**: 488–501.

Eisler I, Le Grange D and Asen E (2003) Family interventions. In: J Treasure, U Schmidt and E van Furth (eds), *Handbook of Eating Disorders* (2e). John Wiley & Sons, Chichester, pp 291–310.

Fairburn C and Harrison P (2003) Eating disorders. *The Lancet*, **361**: 407–16.

First M, Pincus H, Levine J, Williams J, Ustun B and Peele R (2004) Clinical utility as a criterion for revising psychiatric diagnoses. *American Journal of Psychiatry*, **161**: 946–54.

***Fisher M (2003) The course and outcome of EDs in adults and in adolescents: a review. *Adolescent Medicine*, **14**: 149–58.
This is a helpful review of follow-up studies of adults and adolescents, the results of which are summarized and presented separately.

Golden N (2003) Osteopenia and osteoporosis in anorexia nervosa. *Adolescent Medicine*, **14**: 97–108.

***Golden N and Meyer W (2004) Nutritional rehabilitation of anorexia nervosa. Goals and dangers. *International Journal of Adolescent Medicine and Health*, **16**: 131–44.
A comprehensive overview of the often difficult process of refeeding young patients with AN by experienced adolescent medicine clinicians.

***Gowers S and Bryant-Waugh R (2004) Management of child and adolescent EDs: the current evidence base and future directions. *Journal of Child Psychology and Psychiatry*, **45**: 63–83.
A review of the current evidence base and its implications for the management of EDs in children and adolescents.

Gowers S and Smyth B (2004) The impact of a motivational assessment interview on initial response to treatment in adolescent AN. *European Eating Disorders Review*, **12**: 87–93.

Gusella J, Clark S and van Roosmalen E (2004) Body image self-evaluation colouring lens: comparing the ornamental and instrumental views of adolescent girls with EDs. *European Eating Disorders Review*, **12**: 223–9.

Halvorsen I, Andersen A and Heyerdahl S (2004) Good outcome of anorexia nervosa after systematic treatment: intermediate to long term follow-up of a representative county sample. *European Child and Adolescent Psychiatry*, **13**: 295–306.

Hebebrand J, Casper R, Treasure T and Schweiger U (2004) The need to revise the diagnostic criteria for anorexia nervosa. *Journal of Neural Transmission*, **111**: 827–40.

Heer M, Mika C, Grzella I, Heuseen N and Herpetz Dahlman B (2004) Bone turnover during inpatient nutritional therapy and outpatient follow up in patients with AN compared with that in healthy control subjects. *American Journal of Clinical Nutrition*, **80**: 774–81.

Holtkamp K, Hebebrand J and Herpertz–Dahlman B (2004) The contribution of anxiety and food restriction on physical activity levels in acute AN. *International Journal of Eating Disorders*, **36**: 163–71.

Isnard P, Michel G, Frelut M–L, Vila G, Falissard B, Naja W, Navarro J, Mouren-Simeoni M-C (2003) Binge eating and psychopathology in severely obese adolescents. *International Journal of Eating Disorders*, **34**: 235–43.

Karwautz A, Nobis G, Haidvogl M, Wagner G, Hafferl-Gattermayer A, Wöber-Bingöl C and Friedrich M (2003) Perceptions of family relationships in adolescents with anorexia nervosa and their unaffected sisters. *European Child and Adolescent Psychiatry*, **12**: 128–35.

Kendall R and Jablensky A (2003) Distinguishing between the validity and utility of psychiatric diagnoses. *American Journal of Psychiatry*, **160**: 4–12.

Krautter T and Lock J (2004) Treatment of adolescent anorexia nervosa using manualized family-based treatment. *Clinical Case Studies*, **3**: 107–23.

Kreipe R and Yussman S (2003) The role of the primary care practitioner in the treatment of eating disorders. *Adolescent Medicine*, **14**: 133–47.

Le Grange D, Lock J and Dymek M (2003) Family-based therapy for adolescent with bulimia nervosa. *American Journal of Psychotherapy*, **67**: 237–51.

Le Grange D, Binford R and Loeb K (2005) Manualized family based treatment for AN: a case series. *Journal of the American Academy of Child and Adolescent Psychiatry*, **44**: 41–6.

Linscheid T and Butz C (2003) Anorexia nervosa and bulimia nervosa. In: M Roberts (ed), *Handbook of Pediatric Psychology* (3e). Guilford Press, New York, pp 636–51.

Lock J and Le Grange D (2005) *Help Your Teenager Beat an ED*. Guilford Press, New York.

Lock J and Litt I (2003) What predicts maintenance of weight for adolescents medically hospitalized for anorexia nervosa? *Eating Disorders: The Journal of Treatment and Prevention*, **11**: 1–7.

Marcus M and Kalarchian M (2003) Binge eating in children and adolescents. *International Journal of Eating Disorders*, **34**: S47–S57.

Milos G, Spindler A, Schnyder U, Martz J, Hoek H and Willi J (2004) Incidence of severe anorexia nervosa in Switzerland: 40 years of development. *International Journal of Eating Disorders*, **35**: 250–8.

NICE (National Institute for Clinical Excellence) (2004) *Eating Disorders: core interventions in the treatment and management of anorexia nervosa, bulimia nervosa and related eating disorders*. British Psychological Society and Gaskell, London, CG9.

Nicholls D and Bryant-Waugh R (2003) Children and young adolescents. In: J Treasure, U Schmidt and E van Furth (eds), *Handbook of Eating Disorders* (2e). John Wiley & Sons, Chichester, pp 415–33.

O'Herlihy A, Worrall A, Lelliott P, Jaffa T, Mears A, Banerjee S and Hill P (2004) Characteristics of the residents of in-patient child and adolescent mental health services in England and Wales. *Clinical Child Psychology and Psychiatry*, **9**: 579–88.

Okon D, Greene A and Smith JE (2003) Family interactions predict intraindividual symptom variation for adolescents with bulimia. *International Journal of Eating Disorders*, **34**: 450–7.

Råstam M, Gillberg C and Wentz E (2003) Outcome of teenage onset AN in a Swedish community based sample. *European Child and Adolescent Psychiatry*, **12 Suppl 1**: 78–90.

***Rome E, Ammerman S, Rosen D, Keller R, Lock J, Mammel K, O'Toole J, Mitchell Rees J, Sanders M, Sawyer S, Schneider M, Sigel E and Silber T (2003) Children and adolescents with eating disorders: the state of the art. *Pediatrics*, **111**: 98–108.
A helpful overview of a wide range of important aspects of managing young people with EDs put together by an experienced multidisciplinary panel of authors.

Rosen D (2003) Eating disorders in children and young adolescents: etiology, classification, clinical features, and treatment. *Adolescent Medicine*, **14**: 49–59.

Royal Australian and New Zealand College of Psychiatrists (2004) Australian and New Zealand clinical practice guidelines for the treatment of anorexia nervosa. *Australian and New Zealand Journal of Psychiatry*, **38**: 659–70.

Sigman G (2003) Eating disorders in children and adolescents. *Pediatric Clinics of North America*, **50**: 1139–77.

Swenne I (2004) Weight requirements for return of menses in teenage girls with eating disorders, weight loss and secondary amenorrhea. *Acta Paediatrica*, **93**: 11.

Tan J, Hope T and Stewart A (2003) Competence to refuse treatment in AN. *International Journal of Law and Psychiatry*, **26**: 697–707.

Wentz E, Mellström D, Gillberg C, Sundh V, Gillberg C and Råstam M (2003) Bone density 11 years after AN onset in a controlled study of 39 cases. *International Journal of Eating Disorders*, **34**: 314–18.

Wonderlich S, Mitchell J, de Zwaan M and Steiger H (eds) (2005) Academy for Eating Disorders. *Eating Disorders Review. Part 1*. Radcliffe Publishing, Oxford.

9

Treatment of bulimia nervosa

Christopher G Fairburn

Abstract

Objectives of review. To identify advances in the treatment of bulimia nervosa (BN).

Summary of recent findings. The NICE systematic review provides the best appraisal of what has been learned from the research on the treatment of BN, and the accompanying NICE guideline provides impartial evidence-derived recommendations regarding patient management. It is clear that a specific form of cognitive–behavior therapy (CBT) is the leading treatment for BN although its effectiveness needs to be enhanced. Early behavior change in treatment is a potent and reliable predictor of outcome. Managing these patients in primary care is difficult and the results are modest. It appears that self-help is of limited value.

Future directions. There is a need to develop more effective treatments for BN. Research on adolescents is required since it cannot be assumed that findings obtained with adults will apply to younger patients. There is also a need for 'effectiveness' research in which treatments are evaluated under conditions that approximate those existing in routine clinical practice.

Introduction

This paper is concerned with conceptual and practical advances in the treatment of bulimia nervosa (BN), the focus being on papers published in 2003 and 2004.

Literature review

The NICE systematic review and guideline

Bulimia nervosa has been the subject of treatment research for over 20 years and more than 70 randomized controlled trials (RCTs) have been conducted. Characterizing exactly what has, and has not, been learned from such a large body of research is not straightforward. Conventionally this has been done in the form of 'narrative reviews' in which the authors describe and distil the research findings, an example being the review by Wilson and Fairburn (2002). Although such reviews are often of value, they are vulnerable to multiple forms of bias. To reduce the opportunities for bias there has been a move towards conducting 'systematic reviews' in which a standardized approach is taken to the identification of all relevant studies and the synthesis of their findings. Recently several systematic reviews have been published on the treatment of BN (e.g. Nakash-Eisikovits *et al.* 2002; Thompson-Brenner *et al.* 2003; National Collaborating Centre for Mental Health 2004), the NICE review being the most rigorous (Wilson and Shafran 2005).

NICE is the acronym for the National Institute for Clinical Excellence, an organization established in England and Wales for generating evidence-based guidelines for the management of clinical problems across the whole of medicine. What is distinctive about NICE guidelines is that they are derived in an operational and impartial way from a specially commissioned systematic review. The NICE guideline on eating disorders (ED) was published in 2004 (National Collaborating Centre for Mental Health 2004) and it provides the best synthesis and analysis of what has emerged from the research on the treatment of BN (up to early 2004). In essence, three main conclusions were drawn, each accompanied by a treatment recommendation.

1. The leading form of treatment for BN is a specific form of cognitive–behavior therapy (CBT–BN) (Fairburn *et al.* 1993). This involves 16–20 one-to-one treatment sessions over four to five months. There is strong research support for this treatment. Indeed, such is the strength of the evidence that NICE recommended that 'Cognitive behavior therapy for bulimia nervosa, a specifically adapted form of cognitive behavior therapy, should be offered to adults with bulimia nervosa' across the National Health Service (NHS).
2. Interpersonal psychotherapy (IPT) is an alternative to CBT–BN and one that involves about the same amount of therapist contact (Fairburn 1997). However, IPT has considerably less empirical support than CBT–BN and takes up to 12 months longer to achieve equivalent effects. NICE recommended that 'Interpersonal psychotherapy should be considered as an alternative to

cognitive behavior therapy, but patients should be informed it takes eight to 12 months to achieve results comparable to cognitive behavior therapy'.

3. Antidepressant drugs and certain self-help programs (preferably used with some form of professional support) both have some efficacy and are relatively straightforward to implement. However, the evidence suggests that few patients make a full and lasting response to either treatment. NICE recommended that these treatments be viewed as possible first steps in management. NICE further specified that fluoxetine was the antidepressant drug of choice (at a dose of 60 mg daily) and that its beneficial effects would be rapidly apparent.

Cognitive–behavior therapy

Group versus individual CBT–BN

Most studies of CBT–BN have delivered the treatment in an individual one-to-one format in line with the original report on the treatment. Group versions of CBT–BN have been evaluated but the treatments studied have differed from CBT–BN in their strategies and procedures, making it impossible to draw conclusions about the relative effectiveness of group versus individual forms of the treatment. In principle this problem was addressed by Chen and colleagues (2003), who compared group and individual versions of the same form of CBT–BN, the two treatments being matched for intensity and duration. Sixty patients were randomized to the two treatments, 44 of whom completed treatment. Overall, the two treatments did not differ statistically in their effects although there was a trend for rates of cessation from binge eating and purging to be higher with the individual form of the treatment. Unfortunately Chen *et al.*'s study was compromised by its limited power and the fact that the same person conducted the treatments and the assessments. Further RCTs with this design are needed.

Predictors of response to CBT–BN

Knowing what predicts response to treatment is of clinical value since it can aid decision making. It can also enhance understanding of the ways in which treatments work. Attempts to identify predictors of treatment outcome in BN have yielded inconsistent findings. This is probably due to the use of small and heterogeneous patient samples, varying definitions and measures of outcome, and patients' exposure to different forms of treatment.

Recently Agras and colleagues (2000) reported that early behavior change in treatment was a strong predictor of immediate post-treatment response to CBT–BN. This finding was of interest since it came from a large well-conducted multisite study. Fairburn and colleagues (2004) have since replicated and extended this finding using data from a sizeable RCT. As in the Agras *et al.* study, it was found that from among a wide range of potential predictor variables, early behavior change was the best predictor of post-treatment response. In addition, it emerged that early behavior change also predicted patients' state eight months after the end of treatment (i.e. more than 12 months after the behavior change occurred), reinforcing the clinical importance of the finding.

'Relapse' following CBT–BN

Recently it was reported that CBT–BN was associated with a high rate of relapse post treatment. Halmi and colleagues (2002) found that of 48 patients who had ceased to binge eat and purge at the end of treatment, 44% had relapsed within four months. It has since been clarified that their definition of 'relapse' was a somewhat crude research one (i.e. any binge eating or purging whatsoever over the past four weeks) rather than the return of a problem of clinical magnitude. In the context of clarifying this point, Halmi and colleagues (2003) concluded that their findings 'definitely support rather than undermine the standing of CBT as a potent treatment for bulimia nervosa'.

More or less the same sample was the subject of a relapse prevention RCT in which patients were randomized either to the offer of limited additional treatment if they felt it was required or to routine research reassessments (Mitchell *et al.* 2004). The goal was to evaluate a brief intervention designed to nip potential relapses in the bud. Intriguingly, none of the patients took up this offer even though 37% 'relapsed' as defined above. The authors offer various explanations for this finding, an especially plausible one being that the participants did not want to admit to having further problems. What is also important to stress is that many of these relapses were not of clinical severity, so the patients might not have felt a need for further treatment.

Exposure with response prevention

In the 1980s and 1990s various forms of exposure with response prevention (ERP) were evaluated as treatments for BN, either as interventions in their own right or as adjuncts to CBT–BN. In one of the most recent studies of ERP, 135 patients first received an eight-session adaptation of CBT–BN followed either by one or other of two versions of ERP or by relaxation training (Bulik *et al.* 1998). It was found that at the end of treatment and over a 12-month follow-up period neither form of ERP conveyed any advantage over brief CBT–BN followed by relaxation training. The authors concluded that 'The present study strongly supports the efficacy of CBT for bulimia nervosa but offers little support for the inclusion of formal exposure with response prevention treatment packages'. Carter *et al.* (2003a) recently conducted a three-year follow-up of these patients and once again no between-group differences were found.

Mechanisms of action of CBT–BN

Investigating how treatments work is no simple matter. Change is generally rapid and multiple interacting processes are operating. Spangler and colleagues (2004) attempted to investigate the mechanisms of action of CBT–BN using hierarchical linear curve models. Unfortunately, interpreting their findings is difficult, not least because the direction of effects was unclear. Readers interested in the general subject of treatment mediators and moderators are recommended the conceptual paper by Kraemer and colleagues (2002).

Pharmacotherapy

Pharmacological treatment in primary care

As is evident from the findings of the NICE systematic review, pharmacotherapy (specifically treatment with antidepressant medication) is less effective than CBT–BN and doubts remain over how well the changes are maintained. Having said this, drug treatment has one distinct advantage over psychological treatment: it is much easier to disseminate. Of particular interest therefore is the impact of pharmacotherapy in primary care. Walsh and colleagues (2004) addressed this topic in an effectiveness RCT based in two primary care settings. Ninety-one patients were randomized to fluoxetine alone (60 mg daily), placebo alone, fluoxetine plus guided self-help, or placebo plus guided self-help–all delivered over 16 weeks. The findings were salutary. Most patients (69%) did not complete treatment; there was no evidence of any benefit from the self-help program; and while fluoxetine was associated with a greater reduction in the frequency of binge eating and vomiting than placebo, the extent of the improvement was modest. Walsh *et al.* concluded that 'The problems of non-compliance, the lack of evidence for utility of guided self-help, and limited impact of fluoxetine also suggest that early referral to a speciality clinic should be strongly considered for patients with bulimia nervosa seen in primary care settings'.

Fluvoxamine

The findings from a large RCT involving the antidepressant drug fluvoxamine have long been awaited. Schmidt and colleagues (2004) are to be congratulated on obtaining the data and presenting the findings, albeit in outline. The study had a complex design in which 267 patients were randomized to fluvoxamine or placebo, or fluvoxamine then placebo, combined with three different intensities of psychological support, all provided over one year. Somewhat surprisingly, fluvoxamine proved to be no more effective than placebo in both the short and long term and, disturbingly, its use was associated with a high rate of adverse effects, some of which were serious (grand mal seizures). The reason why fluvoxamine was ineffective is not clear, given that most antidepressant drugs seem to have an 'antibulimic' effect, but one possibility is that the dose was too low (range 50 mg to 300 mg; no further details given), although a higher dose might have been associated with even more adverse effects.

Sertraline

In contrast, Milano and colleagues (2004) found that sertraline (100 mg daily) was statistically superior to placebo in reducing the frequency of binge eating and purging. However, this was a small short-term RCT involving the treatment of just 20 patients. No serious adverse effects were observed. Treatment effects of this type and scale have been observed with many other antidepressant drugs.

Topiramate

Topiramate is an antiepileptic drug that is associated with appetite suppression and weight loss. It has recently been investigated as a treatment for BN in an RCT involving 69 (highly selected) patients treated for 10 weeks. The median dose was 100 mg daily (range 25 to 400 mg daily). Topiramate proved to be more effective than placebo in its effects on binge eating and purging and on measures of psychosocial impairment (Hedges *et al.* 2003; Hoopes *et al.* 2003), and the drug was well tolerated. The magnitude of the drug effect was no different from that seen with antidepressant medication.

Genotype and drug response

In a six-week single-blind RCT involving the randomization of 91 patients to four different selective serotonin reuptake inhibitors (SSRIs)–fluvoxamine, fluoxetine, citalopram, paroxetine–or placebo, Erzegovesi and colleagues (2004) examined whether drug response was predicted by allelic variation in the promoter region of the serotonin transporter gene. It was not. The authors claimed that their data also provided evidence of 'substantial equivalence' among the four SSRIs, but as this was not an equivalence trial this conclusion is questionable.

Self-help

Self-help in primary care

Like pharmacotherapy, self-help is a readily disseminated form of treatment. Its effectiveness in primary care therefore needs to be studied. To date there have been two RCTs of self-help in this setting. The study by Walsh and colleagues (2004) was considered earlier in the context of pharmacotherapy studies. It found that guided self-help was associated with poor compliance and few beneficial effects. A likely explanation is that this was a true effectiveness trial conducted under 'field' conditions. Thus the clinical setting was not one that lent itself to the implementation of a psychological intervention, not least because the nurses who 'facilitated' the self-help programme were in an unfamiliar role.

It is difficult to draw conclusions from the second primary care RCT. Sixty-four patients who had been referred for specialist treatment were randomized either to receive whatever treatment the specialist clinic offered or to guided self-help overseen by their family doctor (Durand and King 2003). At six and 12 months post randomization it was found that both groups of patients had improved and there were no statistically significant differences between them. The authors concluded that patients with BN can be treated in general practice. This conclusion, which runs counter to that of Walsh and colleagues (2004), presupposes that the comparison specialist treatment was representative of good clinical practice. In reality the specialist treatment fell far short of this standard since the mean number of sessions that the patients attended was less than five. The utility of this comparison condition is therefore open to question. This objection would be outweighed by evidence that the patients in the two conditions had a good outcome, but this appears not to have been the case. This study therefore shows that inadequate treatment at a specialist clinic and guided self-help in general practice are both unsatisfactory.

Other applications of self-help

Self-help has a variety of other potential uses, two of which have been explored in recent RCTs. Carter and colleagues (2003b) evaluated the effectiveness of self-help as a treatment for patients on a waiting list for specialist treatment. Eighty-five such patients were randomized to one of three eight-week conditions: remaining on the waiting list, a cognitive–behavioral self-help program for BN, or an assertiveness self-help program. Neither of the self-help interventions was accompanied by external support. Patients in all three conditions improved in terms of binge eating and purging but the changes were modest in scale and there was no effect of treatment condition. Nor were there parallel changes in other ED features or general psychiatric symptoms. It therefore seems that the two self-help programs were of little value in this context.

Bailer and colleagues (2004) evaluated an extended form of guided self-help involving 18 weekly sessions. The usual number is about eight. The sessions were overseen by junior residents in psychiatry and each lasted no longer than 20 minutes. The comparison condition was a form of group CBT–BN involving 18 90-minute group sessions held at weekly intervals. The outcome at the end of treatment was poor in both treatment conditions with just 8% and 12% of those randomized to self-help and group CBT–BN, respectively, ceasing to binge eat and purge. The equivalent figures at follow-up were somewhat better at 15% and 23%, but these data are difficult to interpret since over half the patients had by then received additional treatment. Another complicating factor is that the two treatment groups differed at baseline in their rates of current depression, current antidepressant use and lifetime histories of depression and attempted suicide, all of which were more common among those who received group CBT–BN. Overall, it is difficult to draw conclusions from this study.

Summary of important findings

1. The NICE systematic review and guideline provide the best synthesis and appraisal of what has been learned from the research on the treatment of BN and its implications for patient management.
2. CBT–BN is the leading treatment for BN.
3. The relative effectiveness of group versus individual CBT–BN remains unknown.
4. Early behavior change in treatment is a potent and reliable predictor of patients' short- and longer term outcome.
5. Managing these patients in primary care is difficult and the results are modest.
6. Sertraline and topiramate, but not fluvoxamine, may have merit as alternatives to fluoxetine as pharmacological treatments for BN.
7. Self-help (guided or 'pure') appears to be of limited value in the treatment of this disorder.

Clinical implications

The NICE guideline (summarized earlier) identifies in an impartial and objective way the clinical implications of the treatment research to date. The primacy of CBT–BN in the management of BN is clear. The NICE guidance is now being implemented across England and Wales but whether it will have an impact elsewhere remains to be seen. It is of interest to compare both in form and substance the NICE guideline with that of the American Psychiatric Association (Wilson and Shafran 2005).

A finding of clinical importance is that early change in treatment is a potent and reliable predictor of outcome. At present it is not possible to determine whether it is the type of patient who changes early who has a good prognosis, or whether it is the behavior change itself that predicts outcome, or both. Nevertheless, the finding suggests that the first weeks in treatment are crucial and that particular effort should be made to maximize early behavior change. It also suggests that patients who have not made significant changes early on may need additional help (over and above that provided by CBT–BN) if they are to achieve a good outcome.

Overall, the research is consistent in supporting the notion that BN is difficult to treat. Claims otherwise should be viewed with suspicion. It is difficult to escape the conclusion that BN is best managed in specialist settings using evidence-based forms of treatment.

Whilst CBT–BN is the most potent treatment for BN, it results in less than half the patients making a full and lasting recovery (National Collaborating Centre for Mental Health 2004). More effective treatments are therefore needed. Wilson (2005) considers three options in this regard: augmenting CBT–BN with some form of pharmacotherapy; integrating CBT–BN with some other form of psychotherapy; and somehow enhancing the effectiveness of the existing form of CBT–BN. Wilson concludes that the third option is most likely to bear fruit, highlighting Fairburn and colleagues' (2003) new 'enhanced' form of CBT (CBT–E). CBT–E differs from CBT–BN in five main ways. First, there is greater emphasis on achieving early behavior change. Second, there is a formal assessment of progress three weeks into treatment to allow the identification of emerging obstacles to change, treatment then being adjusted to address these obstacles. Third, there is far greater emphasis on modifying these patients' over-evaluation of shape and weight and its expressions (e.g. body checking, body avoidance and 'feeling fat'). Fourth, the treatment branches out, as needed, from the specific psychopathology of BN to address four commonly encountered barriers to change (i.e. mood intolerance, clinical perfectionism, core low self-esteem and interpersonal difficulties). Lastly, and perhaps most controversially, the treatment has been adapted to make it suitable for all forms of ED rather than just BN.

CBT-E is currently under evaluation at various centers and preliminary data suggest that it shows promise both as a more effective treatment for BN and as a treatment for patients with the common DSM–IV diagnosis 'eating disorder not otherwise specified' (Fairburn 2004; Fairburn and Bohn 2005). Its value as a treatment for anorexia nervosa is unclear.

Future directions

There are several priorities. First and foremost, there is a need to develop more effective treatments for BN. The current rate of response is not satisfactory. CBT–E is one attempt in this regard; others are needed. Second, research on adolescents is required since it cannot be assumed that findings obtained with adults will apply to younger patients. Third, there is a need for 'effectiveness' research in which treatments are evaluated under conditions that approximate to those existing in routine clinical practice.

Acknowledgments

I am grateful to the Wellcome Trust for their support (grant 046386). I am also grateful to Zafra Cooper and Roz Shafran for their thoughts on this paper.

Corresponding author: Christopher G Fairburn, Oxford University, Department of Psychiatry, Warneford Hospital, Oxford OX3 7JX, UK. Email: credo@medicine. ox.ac.uk

References

References included from the targeted review years are preceded by one asterisk. References preceded by three asterisks are of particular significance. The significance is explained by a short commentary following the complete reference.

Agras WS, Crow SJ, Halmi KA, Mitchell JE, Wilson GT and Kraemer HC (2000) Outcome predictors for the cognitive behavior treatment of bulimia nervosa: Data from a multisite study. *American Journal of Psychiatry*, **157**: 1302–08.

*Bailer U, de Zwaan M, Leisch F, Strnad A, Lennkh-Wolfsberg C, El Giamal N *et al*. (2004) Guided self-help versus cognitive-behavioral group therapy in the treatment of bulimia nervosa. *International Journal of Eating Disorders*, **35**: 522–37.

Bulik CM, Sullivan PF, Carter FA, McIntosh VV and Joyce PR (1998) The role of exposure with response prevention in the cognitive–behavioral therapy for bulimia nervosa. *Psychological Medicine*, **28**: 611–23.

*Carter FA, McIntosh VVW, Joyce PR, Sullivan PF and Bulik CM (2003a) Role of exposure with response prevention in cognitive–behavioral therapy for bulimia nervosa: Three-year follow-up results. *International Journal of Eating Disorders*, **33**: 127–35.

*Carter JC, Olmsted MP, Kaplan AS, McCabe RE, Mills JS and Aime A (2003b) Self-help for bulimia nervosa: A randomized controlled trial. *American Journal of Psychiatry*, **160**: 973–8.

*Chen E, Touyz SW, Beumont PJV, Fairburn CG, Griffiths R, Butow P *et al*. (2003) Comparison of group and individual cognitive–behavioral therapy for patients with bulimia nervosa. *International Journal of Eating Disorders*, **33**: 241–54.

*Durand MA and King M (2003) Specialist treatment versus self-help for bulimia nervosa: A randomised controlled trial in general practice. *British Journal of General Practice*, **53**: 371–7.

*Erzegovesi S, Riboldi C, Di Bella D, Di Molfetta D, Mapelli F, Negri B *et al*. (2004) Bulimia nervosa, 5-HTTLPR polymorphism and treatment response to four SSRIs – A single-blind study. *Journal of Clinical Psychopharmacology*, **24**: 680–2.

Fairburn CG (1997) Interpersonal psychotherapy for bulimia nervosa. In: DM Garner and PE Garfinkel (eds), *Handbook of Treatment for Eating Disorders*. Guilford Press, New York, pp 278–94.

*Fairburn CG (2004) *On the relationship between clinical research and clinical practice*. Keynote address, Annual Conference of the Academy for Eating Disorders, Orlando, April.

Fairburn CG and Bohn K (2005) Eating disorder NOS (EDNOS): An example of the troublesome 'not otherwise specified' (NOS) category in DSM–IV. *Behaviour Research and Therapy*, **43**: 691–701.

Fairburn CG, Marcus MD and Wilson GT (1993) Cognitive–behavioral therapy for binge eating and bulimia nervosa: A comprehensive treatment manual. In: CG Fairburn and GT Wilson (eds), *Binge Eating: nature, assessment and treatment*. Guilford Press, New York, pp 361–404.

*Fairburn CG, Cooper Z and Shafran R (2003) Cognitive behavior therapy for eating disorders: A 'transdiagnostic' theory and treatment. *Behaviour Research and Therapy*, **41**: 509–28.

***Fairburn CG, Agras WS, Walsh BT, Wilson GT and Stice E (2004) Prediction of outcome in bulimia nervosa by early change in treatment. *American Journal of Psychiatry*, **161**: 2322–4.

Agras and colleagues' (2000) reported that early behavior change during CBT–BN was a strong predictor of immediate post-treatment outcome. This paper describes a large-scale replication of the finding. It emerged that early behavior change also predicted patients' state eight months after the end of treatment, highlighting the clinical importance of the finding.

Halmi KA, Agras WS, Mitchell J, Wilson GT, Crow S, Bryson SW *et al.* (2002) Relapse predictors of patients with bulimia nervosa who achieved abstinence through cognitive behavioral therapy. *Archives of General Psychiatry*, **59**: 1105–09.

*Halmi K, Agras S, Mitchell J, Wilson T and Crow S (2003) Relapse in bulimia nervosa – Reply. *Archives of General Psychiatry*, **60**: 850–1.

*Hedges DW, Reimherr FW, Hoopes SP, Rosenthal NR, Kamin M, Karim R *et al.* (2003) Treatment of bulimia nervosa with topiramate in a randomized, double-blind, placebo-controlled trial, Part 2: Improvements in psychiatric measures. *Journal of Clinical Psychiatry*, **64**: 1449–54.

*Hoopes SP, Reimherr FW, Hedges DW, Rosenthal NR, Kamin M, Karim R *et al.* (2003) Treatment of bulimia nervosa with topiramate in a randomized, double-blind, placebo-controlled trial, Part 1: Improvements in binge and purge measures. *Journal of Clinical Psychiatry*, **64**: 1335–41.

Kraemer HC, Wilson GT, Fairburn CG and Agras WS (2002) Mediators and moderators of treatment effects in randomized clinical trials. *Archives of General Psychiatry*, **59**: 877–83.

*Milano W, Petrella C, Sabatino C and Capasso A (2004) Treatment of bulimia nervosa with sertraline: A randomized controlled trial. *Advances in Therapy*, **21**: 232–7.

***Mitchell JE, Agras WS, Wilson GT, Halmi K, Kraemer H and Crow S (2004) A trial of a relapse prevention strategy in women with bulimia nervosa who respond to cognitive–behavior therapy. *International Journal of Eating Disorders*, **35**: 549–55.

This paper describes a relapse prevention RCT in which patients who had responded to CBT–BN were randomized either to the offer of limited additional treatment if they felt it was required or to routine research reassessments. Intriguingly, none of the patients took up this offer. This finding raises several important issues including what constitutes a 'relapse' of clinical magnitude.

Nakash-Eisikovits O, Dierberger A and Westen D (2002) A multidimensional meta-analysis of pharmacotherapy for bulimia nervosa: Summarizing the range of outcomes in controlled clinical trials. *Harvard Review of Psychiatry*, **10**: 193–211.

***National Collaborating Centre for Mental Health (2004) *Eating Disorders: core interventions in the treatment and management of anorexia nervosa, bulimia nervosa and related eating disorders*. British Psychological Society and Royal College of Psychiatrists, London.

The NICE guideline on eating disorders provides the best synthesis and analysis of what has emerged from the research on the treatment of bulimia nervosa (up to early 2004) and its implications for patient management.

*Schmidt U, Cooper PJ, Essers H, Freeman CPL, Holland RL, Palmer RL *et al.* (2004) Fluvoxamine and graded psychotherapy in the treatment of bulimia nervosa – A randomized, double-blind, placebo-controlled, multicenter study of short-term and long-term pharmacotherapy combined with a stepped care approach to psychotherapy. *Journal of Clinical Psychopharmacology*, **24**: 549–52.

***Spangler DL, Baldwin SA and Agras WS (2004) An examination of the mechanisms of action in cognitive behavioral therapy for bulimia nervosa. *Behavior Therapy*, **35**: 537–60.

This paper describes an attempt to study the mechanisms of action of CBT–BN. Readers interested in the general subject of treatment mediators and moderators are recommended the conceptual paper by Kraemer and colleagues (2002).

*Thompson-Brenner H, Glass S and Westen D (2003) A multidimensional meta-analysis of psychotherapy for bulimia nervosa. *Clinical Psychology – Science and Practice*, **10**: 269–87.

***Walsh BT, Fairburn CG, Mickley D, Sysko R and Parides MK (2004) Treatment of bulimia nervosa in a primary care setting. *American Journal of Psychiatry*, **161**: 556–61.

This paper describes an 'effectiveness' RCT based in primary care in which fluoxetine alone, placebo alone, fluoxetine plus guided self-help, and placebo plus guided self-help were compared. Compliance was poor and the patients fared badly. The conclusion

drawn is that patients with BN should be referred for specialist treatment rather than managed in primary care.

Wilson GT (2005) Psychological treatment of eating disorders. *Annual Review of Clinical Psychology,* **1**: 439–65.

Wilson GT and Fairburn CG (2002) Treatments for eating disorders. In: PE Nathan and JM Gorman (eds), *A Guide to Treatments that Work* (2e). Oxford University Press, New York, pp 559–592.

Wilson GT and Shafran R (2005) Eating disorders guidelines from NICE. *The Lancet,* **365**: 79–81.

10

Treatment of anorexia nervosa

Katherine A Halmi

Abstract

Objectives of review. The purpose of this review is to provide an update on treatment interventions for anorexia nervosa (AN). These interventions cover psychotherapy, pharmacotherapy, medical management, and psychiatric management.

Summary of recent findings. There are few randomized controlled clinical trials for treatment of AN. A multidimensional treatment including a physician, a psychiatrist, an experienced eating disorder therapist and a registered dietician is recommended. Family therapy for adolescent AN patients is beneficial. Cognitive–behavioral therapy (CBT) is most useful and serotonin reuptake inhibitors are helpful for preventing relapse.

Future directions. There is a problem with AN patients accepting treatment and being motivated to give up their illness. Developing therapeutic strategies that address motivation as well as innovative interventions that may affect the anorectic's sense of confidence and security with interpersonal problems and other life issues are needed. Large, collaborative randomized controlled trials (RCTs) will not give meaningful information if patients refuse to participate and the dropout rate remains high.

Introduction

During 2004 three publications on guidelines for the treatment of anorexia nervosa (AN) were published. The British National Institute for Clinical Excellence (NICE) developed a grading scheme for which all treatment was classified according to an accepted hierarchy of empirical evidence supporting specific treatments. Recommendations were graded A through C, based on the level of associated evidence. Grade A was evidence obtained from a single RCT or a meta-analysis of RCTs. Grade B ranged from evidence obtained from at least one designed controlled study without randomization to evidence obtained from well-designed descriptive studies such as comparative studies, correlational studies and case–control studies. Grade C was evidence obtained from expert committee reports, or opinion and clinical experiences of respected authorities (NICE 2004). The recommendation from this analysis for AN treatment was an overall grade of C because of the very few RCTs. The specific recommendations differ little from the practice guidelines developed by the APA Workgroup (American Psychiatric Association Workgroup 2000). The NICE summary for treating AN patients is as follows:

1. whenever possible these patients should be managed on an outpatient basis, with psychological treatment given by an experienced and competent service that also assesses physical risks;
2. inpatient treatment should be in an experienced setting that can implement refeeding with careful physical monitoring and provide psychosocial interventions;
3. family intervention that directly addresses the eating disorder should be offered to children and adolescents.

An alternative set of guidelines from the Royal Australian and New Zealand College of Psychiatrists (2004) acknowledge that their recommendations necessarily rely on expert opinion and not on controlled trials. They recommend a multidimensional approach to treatment of AN with close attention to medical manifestations and weight restoration. No specific psychotherapy is recommended, but family therapy is mentioned as a valuable part of treatment for children and adolescents. Additional suggestions include that dietary advice be part of all treatment programs, antidepressants may be useful in patients with depressive symptoms, and olanzapine may be useful in attenuating hyperactivity.

The Cochrane Review of six small outpatient psychotherapy trials concluded that no specific psychotherapy approach can be recommended. The authors were puzzled why 'treatment as usual' performed so poorly and why dietary advice alone appeared so unacceptable (high dropout rate). Their conclusion was there is an urgent need for large well-designed trials assessing treatment for AN (Hay *et al.* 2004).

This paper will provide a critical review of the salient treatment literature in the past few years, including psychotherapy, pharmacotherapy, medical management and psychiatric management.

Psychotherapy interventions

Randomized controlled treatment trials are extremely rare for AN. Psycho-therapy for AN in adults draws on psychodynamic, cognitive and systemic theories. Dare *et al*. (2001) assessed the effectiveness of specific psychotherapies in outpatient management of adult patients with AN. Eighty-four AN patients were randomized to one of three specific psychotherapies:

1. one year of social psychoanalytic therapy
2. seven months of cognitive–analytic therapy
3. family therapy for one year
4. low-contact, routine treatment for one year (control group).

At one year there was modest symptomatic improvement in the whole group of patients, with several being significantly undernourished. The three specific psychotherapies showed some benefits over the control treatment.

Another randomized controlled treatment trial assessed two forms of out-patient family intervention for AN (Eisler *et al*. 2000). Forty adolescent AN patients were randomly assigned to conjoint family therapy (CFT) or to sep-arated family therapy (SFT) using a stratified design controlling for levels of critical comments with the Expressed Emotion Index. The therapist conducted both forms of treatment. A marked improvement in nutritional and psycho-logical state occurred across both treatment groups. For those patients with high levels of maternal criticisms towards the patient, the SFT was shown to be superior to the CFT. On a global measure of outcome, the two forms of therapy were associated with equivalent end-of-treatment results.

In a third RCT, 33 patients with AN were randomly assigned to one year of outpatient CBT or nutritional counseling after inpatient hospitalization (Pike *et al*. 2003). The group receiving nutritional counseling relapsed significantly earlier and at a higher rate than the group receiving CBT (53% versus 22%). The overall treatment failure rate, relapse and dropping out combined, was signifi-cantly lower for CBT (22%) than for nutritional counseling (73%). The criteria for good outcome were met by significantly more of the patients receiving CBT (44%) than nutritional counseling (7%). This study showed that CBT was markedly more effective than nutritional counseling for improving outcome and preventing relapse. It should be noted that these patients entered the out-patient randomization after being hospitalized in a state-supported research unit where patients were not subjected to managed care policies regarding treatment choice. Considering the fact that these patients entered the post-hospitalization randomization within a normal weight range and a significant psychological improvement, the 22% failure rate of CBT is of some concern.

Three different forms of behavior therapy were compared in a Japanese inpatient treatment setting (Okamoto *et al*. 2002). In this comparison seven patients received activity restriction therapy, seven received a token economy therapy with activity restriction, and 21 received activity restriction therapy with liquid formula in the early stages of hospitalization and establishment of a target weight during the later stages of hospitalization. The liquid formula with activity restriction was the most effective program with regard to both the amount and rate of increase of BMI measured at the end of hospitalization and six months after discharge. The authors suggested the effectiveness of the latter program was due to the use of liquid formula, the setting of a target weight at a later stage of hospitalization, and the release of activity restriction based on weight gain.

Pharmacotherapy intervention

Randomized, placebo-controlled, double-blind pharmacological treatment trials in AN are extremely limited. All guidelines recommend that medication should not be used as the sole or primary treatment for AN. The most recent RCTs had been conducted with serotonin reuptake inhibitors. Although the study by Attia *et al.* (1998) was conducted seven years ago it is worth mentioning, because it was the only randomized, placebo-controlled double-blind study of an adequate sample size assessing fluoxetine for the inpatient treatment of AN. The rationale for testing fluoxetine on these patients was that they frequently exhibit depression and symptoms of obsessive–compulsive disorder (OCD). Thirty-one women with AN received up to 60 mg per day of fluoxetine for seven weeks. They were treated on a clinical research unit and received supportive psychotherapy as well as being in a structured environment. After seven weeks there was no significant difference in clinical outcome on any measure between patients receiving fluoxetine and those on placebo. Thus, fluoxetine does not appear to add any significant benefit to the inpatient treatment of AN.

In another placebo-controlled double-blind fluoxetine treatment study of AN, 35 patients were randomly assigned to fluoxetine or placebo after inpatient weight gain and were observed as outpatients for one year. Ten of 16 (63%) patients remained on fluoxetine for a year, whereas only three of 19 (16%) remained on placebo for a year. Although this study has serious methodological problems (e.g. in the outpatient phase of the psychotherapy was uncontrolled and occurred in a large variety of sites), there is suggestive evidence that fluoxetine may be useful in preventing relapse in AN patients after weight restoration (Kaye *et al.* 2001).

A pilot study conducted by Fassino *et al.* (2002) randomized 26 AN outpatients to citalopram and 26 to a waiting list control group. Of the 52 subjects in the study, 13 patients dropped out, with 19 subjects actually receiving citalopram and 20 remained in the control group. After three months of treatment, the citalopram group showed a decrease in depression and an improvement of obsessive–compulsive features. Weight gain was similar in the two groups. Citalopram seemed to alleviate depression, obsessive–compulsive symptoms, impulsiveness, and trait anger in these patients.

Two uncontrolled studies suggest olanzapine may be useful in treating AN patients. In a study by Malina *et al.* (2003) 18 AN patients who had received olanzapine were retrospectively questioned about their response. Generally they reported a significant reduction in anxiety, difficulty eating and core eating disorder (ED) symptoms. Powers *et al.* (2002) studied 18 AN patients in an open label study of olanzapine, 10 mg per day. Of the 14 patients who completed the study, 10 gained an average of 8.75 pounds and three of these obtained their ideal bodyweight. The remaining four patients who completed the study lost a mean of 2.25 pounds. These findings are promising with clinically significant weight gain in an outpatient setting during a brief 10-week period.

A single-blind comparison of amisulpride, fluoxetine and clomipramine in restricting AN patients was conducted by Rigerrio *et al.* (2001). This was a single-blind condition in which 13 patients received clomipramine, 10 patients received fluoxetine and 12 patients received amisulpride. Mean dosages were 57.7 mg, 28 mg, and 50 mg, respectively. Patients treated with amisulpride had a significantly greater increase of mean weight compared to the other two drugs. No difference was present in measures of weight phobia, body-image disturbance and amenorrhea.

Finally, an open-controlled trial of sertraline was conducted in 11 restricting AN patients by Santonastaso *et al.* (2001). At the 14-week follow-up, the sertraline group of 11 reported a significantly greater improvement of depressive symptoms, ineffectiveness, lack of enteroceptive awareness and perfectionism when compared to a control group that received no drug and no placebo. Both groups reported a significant improvement in bodyweight. At the 64-week follow-up one patient in the sertraline group and five patients in the control group still had a full diagnosis of an ED. This was an outpatient study and suggests that it may be worthwhile to conduct a larger placebo-controlled double-blind study of sertraline for the treatment of AN. It should be noted that these outpatients also received a multidisciplinary treatment with nutritional counseling and psychotherapy.

Medical management

Medical management is a necessary part of the treatment of AN patients. Advice on medical management is based on the experience of clinicians and not RCTs. It is generally recognized that nutritional rehabilitation programs should establish healthy target weights with a weight gain of two to three pounds a week for inpatient treatment and one pound per week for outpatient programs. Intake levels should usually start at 30–40 kcal/kg per day (approximately 1000–1600 kcal/day) and advance by 500 calories every few days. Patients must be monitored for discarding food, vomiting, or exercising frequently. Medical monitoring during refeeding includes assessment of vital signs, food and fluid intake and output, assessment of electrolytes (including phosphorus) and observation for edema, rapid weight gain with fluid overload, congestive heart failure, constipation, and bloating. For severely malnourished patients less than 70% of standard bodyweight, cardiac monitoring may be necessary. Physical activity should be adapted to the food intake and energy expenditure of the patient. Supplementation or replacement of regular food with liquid food supplements may be very helpful in the initial stages of treatment. Nasogastric feedings may be required in life-threatening circumstances. Parenteral feedings are associated with an infection risk and should be rarely considered only in patients in whom nasogastric feedings are considered hazardous. Forceful interventions should be considered only when the patients are unwilling to cooperate with oral feedings and their physical safety is in danger. During hospitalization, use of liquid formula in the early stages of weight gain with gradual exposure to food and gradual increase in activity can be very effective in inducing weight gain (Okamoto *et al.* 2002).

An RCT was conducted by Birmingham *et al.* (2004) to determine if warming therapy would increase the rate of weight gain in AN patients who were hospitalized for refeeding. This study was done to test the hypothesis that placing AN patients in a warm environment will help them to relax and thus gain weight more easily. This was tested in 21 patients of whom 10 were randomized to a heating vest for three hours a day for 21 days and 11 were randomized to the vest set in an off position. In the 18 completers, there was no difference in the change in BMI. This study did not demonstrate an increase in the rate of weight gain with body temperature warming.

Another RCT study assessed the effect of recombinant human growth hormone (rhGH) for weight gain in hospitalized AN patients. Fifteen adolescent anorexia patients were enrolled in a 28-day randomized, double-blind, placebo-controlled study. The patients received rhGH 0.05 mg/kg subcutaneously or an equivalent volume of placebo daily. Outpatients received a standard refeeding protocol. There were no significant differences in weight gain and length of hospitalization in the two groups (Hill *et al.* 2000).

The impact of high-calorie supplements, in addition to a normal diet, was examined in a study comparing 29 inpatients who received the supplements with 29 inpatients without this substitution. Those who received the supplementation had a more rapid weight gain, a greater weight on discharge, and a shorter therapy duration (Imbierowicv *et al.* 2002).

The use of nutritional supplements to increase the efficacy of fluoxetine in the treatment of AN was studied in a double-blind placebo-controlled manner by Barbarich *et al.* (2004). Twenty-six AN patients received either fluoxetine and a nutritional supplement consisting of tryptophan, vitamins, minerals and essential fatty acids, or fluoxetine and a nutritional placebo. There were no significant differences in weight gain between the two groups. Also there were no mean changes in anxiety or obsessive–compulsive symptoms between groups. These results suggest that supplement strategies are not a substitute for adequate nutrition and are ineffective in increasing the efficacy of fluoxetine in underweight AN patients.

Two studies examined nutritional deficiencies during refeeding of AN patients. A retrospective chart review of 69 AN patients admitted to an inpatient medical unit found 19 (27.5%) patients required phosphorus supplementation. Phosphorus levels dropped to a nadir during the first week of refeeding. The authors recommended daily monitoring of serum phosphorus with supplementation as needed during the first week of hospitalization, especially in those who are severely malnourished (Ornstein *et al.* 2003).

Persistence of nutritional deficiencies after short-term weight recovery in adolescents with AN was studied by Castro *et al.* (2004). In this study hormonal abnormalities reverted to normal after renutrition. There were decreases in folic acid levels and zinc levels increased, but did not reach normal levels. The authors recommended supplementation of folic acid and zinc for AN patients.

Finally, estrogen replacement in AN patients with chronic amenorrhea has not been shown to prevent or reverse bone loss (Grinspoon *et al.* 2002; Golden 2003).

Psychiatric management

There are no adequate RCTs to determine the efficacy of initial treatment intensity or type for AN patients. Some partial hospitalization programs have been found to be effective in direct relation to their intensity; that is, programs with 12 hour, 6 days a week treatment may approach inpatient programs in their effectiveness, whereas programs with fewer hours and fewer days of the week lose effectiveness (Zipfel *et al.* 2002; Olmstead *et al.* 2003).

Various factors such as the patient's specific physiological and psychiatric status, the patient and family's motivation and ability to adhere to a weight gain plan, and personal and local resources determine whether the patient will be hospitalized. For patients whose initial weight falls below 75% of expected weight and even higher for children who are losing weight rapidly, hospitalization is often necessary to assure adequate intake and limit physical activity. Specialized ED units yield better outcome than general psychiatric units because of the specific nursing expertise and more effective protocols (Wolfe and Gimby 2003). A study by Watson *et al.* (2000) suggested that short-term outcomes for involuntarily hospitalized patients are similar to those voluntarily admitted. Comorbid psychiatric disorders such as OCD, severe mood disorder and/or substance dependence require treatment modifications entailing psychiatric medications and psychotherapy.

Summary of important findings

There are few randomized controlled clinical trials to provide guidance for treatment of AN. Systematic open and observational studies suggest that the initial treatment should focus on nutritional rehabilitation. A multidimensional treatment approach should be organized with a physician, a psychiatrist who can manage pharmacological treatment, an experienced ED therapist, and a registered dietician. Controlled studies have shown that family therapy for adolescent AN patients is highly beneficial. There are difficulties in initiating and sustaining psychotherapy for adult AN patients. Cognitive–behavioral therapy is useful and after weight gain is helpful for preventing relapse.

Adding SSRI to refeeding is not helpful until patients reach close to 80% of their target weight, when they may reduce depression and anxiety. For patients who are treatment resistant, it may be necessary to commit them against their will for inpatient treatment when their medical or psychiatric state is threatening. At the present time the best treatment for AN is a multidimensional treatment plan as mentioned above.

Clinical implications

In the past few years a few randomized controlled treatment trials have indicated that family therapy, either in the conjoint form or with separate parental counseling is effective for producing a better outcome in adolescents with AN. Thus, family therapy or counseling in some form or another should be a necessary part of the treatment of adolescents with AN. There is suggestive evidence that CBT is useful in all stages of AN and fluoxetine given after weight gain may be helpful in preventing relapse in adult AN patients. Treatment with an SSRI to reduce depression, anxiety symptoms and obsessive–compulsive features when AN patients are within 80% of target weight, together with psychotherapies including family meetings and cognitive–behavioral principles, are recommended for treating AN patients.

Future directions

There is a serious problem with AN patients accepting treatment and being motivated to give up their illness and follow through with treatment recommendations. Dropout rates in all RCTs are high. It is well documented by experienced clinicians that AN patients are resistant to treatment and following through in a cooperative manner with therapy techniques to change their behavior. One study showed that AN patients who have healthy relationships and perfectionistic self-standards have better prognosis than those who are avoidant, constricted or who have a somewhat chaotic emotional dysregulation (Westen and Harnden-Fisher 2001). Continuing to develop therapies that address motivation may be useful (Geller 2002). Additional innovative interventions may affect the anorectic's interpersonal attachment style (Ward et al. 2000) and the patient's overall sense of attachment to life (Bachar et al. 2002). Large, collaborative RCTs will not give meaningful information if patients refuse to participate and the dropout rate remains high. It is well known that dropout rates with family therapy for adolescent AN patients are significantly lower than those that occur in treatment trials with adult AN patients. Future research must deal with the problems of resistances to treatment and develop innovative techniques to address this issue.

Corresponding author: Katherine A Halmi, Professor of Psychiatry, Weill Cornell Medical College, Director Eating Disorder Program, New York Presbyterian Hospital, Westchester Division, 21 Bloomingdale Road, White Plains, NY 10605, USA. Email: kah29@cornell.edu

References

References preceded by three asterisks are of particular significance. The significance is explained by a short commentary following the complete reference.

American Psychiatric Association Work Group on Eating Disorders (2000) Practice guidelines for the treatment of patients with eating disorders (revision). *American Journal of Psychiatry*, **157(1 Suppl)**: 1–39.

Attia E, Haiman C, Walsh BT and Flater SR (1998) Does fluoxetine augment the inpatient treatment of anorexia nervosa? *American Journal of Psychiatry*, **155**: 548–51.

Bachar E, Latzer Y, Ganetti L, Gur E, Berry EM and Bonne O (2002) Rejection of life in anorectic and bulimic patients. *International Journal of Eating Disorders*, **31**: 43–8.

Barbarich N, McConaha C, Halmi KA, Gendall K, Sunday S, Gaskill J, LaVia M, Frank GK, Brook S, Plotnikov K and Kaye W (2004) Use of nutritional supplements to increase the efficacy of fluoxetine in the treatment of anorexia nervosa. *International Journal of Eating Disorders*, **35**: 10–15.

***Birmingham CL, Gutierrez E, Jona TL and Beumont P (2004) Randomized controlled trial of warming in anorexia nervosa. *International Journal of Eating Disorders*, **35**: 234–8.

This study was of special interest because it was designed in response to a hypothesis based on the idea that AN can be effectively treated by a warm environment. A previous study, which had serious methodological problems, tried to demonstrate that fact. This study, which was conducted with a proper methodology, showed that there was no increase in rate of weight gain with warming.

Castro J, Deulofeu R, Gila A, Puig J and Toro J (2004) Persistence of nutritional deficiencies after short-term weight recovery in adolescents with anorexia nervosa. *International Journal of Eating Disorders*, **35**: 169–78.

Dare C, Eisler I, Russell G, Treasure J and Dodge L (2001) Psychological therapies for adults with anorexia nervosa: Randomized controlled trial of outpatient treatments. *British Journal of Psychiatry*, **178**: 216–21.

***Eisler I, Dare C, Hodes M, Russell G, Dodge E and Lee GD (2000) Family therapy for adolescent anorexia nervosa: The result of a controlled comparison of two family interventions. *Journal of Child Psychology and Psychiatry*, **41**: 727–36.

This study was of special interest because it showed that family therapy given conjointly or separately with parents being counseled separately were equally effective in adolescent AN families. The other interesting outcome in this study was that the patients with high levels of maternal criticism did better in separated family therapy.

Fassino S, Leombruni P, Daga G, Brustolin A, Migliaretti G, Cavallo F and Rovera G (2002) Efficacy of Citalopram in anorexia nervosa: A pilot study. *European Neuropsychopharmacology*, **12**: 453–9.

Geller J (2002) Estimating readiness for change in anorexia nervosa: Company clients, clinicians and research assessors. *International Journal of Eating Disorders*, **31**: 251–60.

Golden N (2003) Osteopenia and osteoporosis in anorexia nervosa. *Adolescent Medicine*, **14**: 97–108.

Grinspoon S, Thomas L, Miller K, Herzog D and Klibanski A (2002) Effects of recombinant human IGH–I and oral contraceptive administration on bone density and anorexia nervosa. *Journal of Clinical and Endocrinological Metabolism*, **87**: 2883–91.

***Hay P, Bacaltchuk J, Caludino A, Ben-Tovim D and Yong PY (2004) Individual psychotherapy in the outpatient treatment of adults with anorexia nervosa (Cochrane Review). In: The Cochrane Library, issue 3. John Wiley & Sons Ltd, Chichester, UK.

This paper is a review based on a very comprehensive literature search and bases its comments on all available RCTs of adult individual outpatient therapy for AN. Only six

RCTs were identified and described. The authors' conclusion was that no specific approach could be recommended from their review but they recommended that dietary advice alone without therapy should not be given.

Hill K, Bucuvalas J, McClain C, Kryscio R, Martini RT, Alfaro M and Maloney M (2000) Pilot study of growth hormone administration during the refeeding of malnourished anorexia nervosa patients. *Journal of Child and Adolescent Psychopharmacology*, **10**: 3–8.

Imbierowicz K, Braks K, Jacoby G, Geiser F, Conrad R, Schilling G and Liedtke R (2002) High-calorie supplements in anorexia treatment. *International Journal of Eating Disorders*, **32**: 135–45.

Kaye WH, Nagata T and Weltzin TE (2001) Double-blind placebo-controlled administration of fluoxetine in restricting and restricting–purging type anorexia nervosa. *Biological Psychiatry*, **49**: 644–52.

Malina A, Gakill J, McConaha C, Frank G, LaVia M, Scholar L and Kaye W (2003) Olanzapine treatment of anorexia nervosa: A retrospective study. *International Journal of Eating Disorders*, **33**: 234–7.

***NICE (National Institute for Clinical Excellence) (2004) Core interventions in the treatment and management of anorexia nervosa, bulimia nervosa and related eating disorders. *Clinical Guidelines, Number 9*. NICE, London, pp 1–15.
This British document developed by a group of ED experts recommends core intervention in the treatment and management of AN, BN and related EDs. Robustness of treatment evidence is rated according to RCTs, open trials or expert opinion.

Okamoto A, Yamashita T and Nagoshi Y (2002) A behavior therapy program combined with liquid nutrition designed for anorexia nervosa. *Psychiatry and Clinical Neuroscience*, **56**: 515–20.

Olmsted M, Kaplan A and Rockert W (2003) Relative efficacy of a 4 day versus a 5 day hospital program. *International Journal of Eating Disorders*, **34**: 441–9.

Ornstein R, Golden NH, Jacobson MS and Shenker IR (2003) Hypophosphatemia during nutritional rehabilitation in anorexia nervosa: Implications for refeeding and monitoring. *Journal of Adolescent Health*, **32**: 83–8.

Pike KM, Walsh BT, Vitousek K, Wilson GT and Bauer J (2003) Cognitive behavior therapy in the post hospitalization treatment of anorexia nervosa. *American Journal of Psychiatry*, **160**: 2046–9.

Powers PS, Santana CA and Bannon YS (2002) Olanzapine in the treatment of anorexia nervosa: An open label trial. *International Journal of Eating Disorders*, **32**: 146–54.

***Royal Australian and New Zealand College of Psychiatrists Clinical Practice Guidelines Team for Anorexia Nervosa (2004) Australian and New Zealand Clinical Practice Guidelines for the Treatment of Anorexia Nervosa. *Australian and New Zealand Journal of Psychiatry*, **38**: 659–70.
These guidelines rely largely on expert opinion and on controlled trials. They contain convenient tables for medical aspects of eating disorders and levels of care.

Ruggiero GM, Laini V, Mauri MC, Ferrari VM, Clemente E, Lugo F, Mantera M and Cavagnini F (2001) A single-blind comparison of amisulpride, fluoxetine and clomipramine in the treatment of restricting anorectics. *Progress in Neuropsychopharmacology and Biological Psychiatry*, **25**: 1049–59.

Santonastaso P, Friederici S and Favaro A (2001) Sertraline in the treatment of restricting anorexia nervosa: An open controlled trial. *Journal of Child and Adolescent Psychopharmacology*, **11**: 143–50.

Ward A, Ramsay R and Treasure J (2000) Attachment research in eating disorders. *British Journal of Medical Psychology*, **73**: 35–51.

Watson TL, Bowers W and Anderson AE (2000) Involuntary treatment of eating disorders. *American Journal of Psychiatry*, **157**: 1806–10.

Westen D and Harnden-Fisher J (2001) Personality profiles in eating disorders: Rethinking the distinction between Axis I and Axis II. *American Journal of Psychiatry*, **158**: 547–62.

Wolfe BE and Gimby LB (2003) Caring for the hospitalized patient with an eating disorder. *Nursing Clinics of North America*, **38**: 75–99.

Zipfel S, Reas DL and Thornton C (2002) Day hospitalization programs for eating disorders: A systematic review of the literature. *International Journal of Eating Disorders*, **31**: 105–17.

Index